Bayer-Symposium III

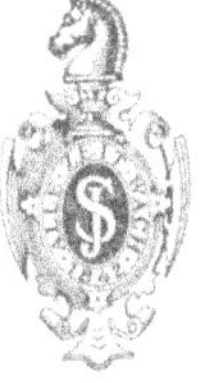

Bacterial Infections

Changes in their Causative Agents
Trends and Possible Basis

Edited by

M. Finland · W. Marget · K. Bartmann

With 53 Figures

Springer-Verlag Berlin · Heidelberg · New York 1971

Professor Maxwell Finland, M.D., Epidemiologist, Department of Health and Hospitals,
Channing Laboratory, Boston City Hospital, Boston, MA 02118/USA

Professor Dr. Walter Marget, Leiter der Abteilung für antimikrobielle Therapie
an der Universitäts-Kinderklinik D-8000 München

Professor Dr. Karl Bartmann, Leiter des Instituts für medizinische Mikrobiologie
der Farbenfabriken Bayer AG, D-5600 Wuppertal-Elberfeld

The editors are indebted to Miss M. L. Chamberlain and Dr. H. Otten
for their valuable assistance

Bayer-Symposium III
held at Grosse Ledder near Cologne, Germany
October 23—27, 1970

ISBN-13: 978-3-642-65269-1   e-ISBN-13: 978-3-642-65267-7
DOI: 10.1007/978-3-642-65267-7

Bayer-Symposium III

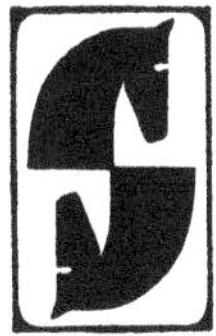

Bacterial Infections

Changes in their Causative Agents
Trends and Possible Basis

Edited by

M. Finland · W. Marget · K. Bartmann

With 53 Figures

Springer-Verlag New York · Heidelberg · Berlin 1971

Professor Maxwell Finland, M.D., Epidemiologist, Department of Health and Hospitals, Channing Laboratory, Boston City Hospital, Boston, MA 02118/USA

Professor Dr. Walter Marget, Leiter der Abteilung für antimikrobielle Therapie an der Universitäts-Kinderklinik D-8000 München

Professor Dr. Karl Bartmann, Leiter des Instituts für medizinische Mikrobiologie der Farbenfabriken Bayer AG, D-5600 Wuppertal-Elberfeld

The editors are indebted to Miss M. L. Chamberlain and Dr. H. Otten for their valuable assistance

Bayer-Symposium III

held at Grosse Ledder near Cologne, Germany

October 23—27, 1970

ISBN-13: 978-3-642-65269-1   e-ISBN-13: 978-3-642-65267-7
DOI: 10.1007/978-3-642-65267-7

Contents

List of Participants

Prof. Dr. K. Bartmann, Farbenfabriken Bayer AG, Institut f. med. Mikrobiologie, D-5600 Wuppertal 1, Friedrich-Ebert-Str. 217—219

Prof. Dr. F. Benazet, Départment de Bactériologie et de Parasitologie, Laboratoires de Recherches, Rhone-Poulence, F-94 Vitry-sur-Seine

Dr. Y.-A. Chabbert, Institut Pasteur, Service de Sensibilité aux Antibiotiques, 25, Rue du Docteur Roux, F-75 Paris XVe

Dr. F. Daschner, Cedars-Sinai Medical Center, 4833 Fountain Avenue, Los Angeles, CA 90029/USA

Prof. Dr. H. Ericsson, Bacteriological Department, Karolinska Sjukhuset, S-Stockholm 60

Prof. M. Finland, Department of Health and Hospitals, Channing Laboratory, Boston City Hospital, 774 Albany Street, Boston, MA 02118/USA

Dr. J. C. Gould, South-Eastern Regional Hospital Board, Central Microbiological Laboratories, Western General Hospital, Crewe Road, GB-Edinburgh, EH4 2XU/Scotland

Prof. Dr. A. von Graevenitz, Yale-New Haven Hospital, 789 Howard Avenue, New Haven, CT 06504/USA

Prof. Dr. O. Gsell, Med. Universitäts-Poliklinik Basel, CH-Basel, Maiengasse 56

Dr. R. I. Holt, Queen Mary's Hospital for Children, Group Laboratories, GB-Carshalton, Surrey

Prof. E. H. Kass, Channing Laboratory, Harvard Medical School, City of Boston Department of Health and Hospitals, 774 Albany Street, Boston, MA 02118/USA

Prof. Dr. H. Knothe, Hygiene-Institut der Universität Frankfurt, D-6000 Frankfurt/M., Paul-Ehrlich-Str. 40

Prof. Dr. G. Linzenmeier, Institut für med. Mikrobiologie, D-43 Essen, Hufelandstraße 55

Dr. E. Lund, Pneumococcus Department, Statens Seruminstitut, Amager Boulevard 80, DK-Kopenhagen S

Prof. Dr. W. Marget, Abt. für antimikrob. Therapie, Universitäts-Kinderklinik München, D-8000 München, Lindwurmstraße 4

Prof. Dr. P. Naumann, Institut f. med. Mikrobiologie und Virologie, Universität Düsseldorf, D-4000 Düsseldorf, Moorenstraße 5

Prof. Dr. G. Pulverer, Hygiene-Institut der Universität Köln, D-5000 Köln-Lindenthal, Fürst-Pückler-Straße 56

Prof. Dr. H. Reber, Universitäts-Klinik Bürgerspital CH-Basel

Prof. R. A. Shooter, Department of Bacteriology, St. Bartholomew's Hospital, GB-London, E.C. 1

Prof. Dr. W. Siegenthaler, Med. Universitäts-Poliklinik, D-5300 Bonn, Wilhelmstraße 35/37

Prof. R. E. O. Williams, St. Mary's Hospital Medical School, Department of Bacteriology, Wright-Fleming Institute, Paddington GB-London, W. 2

P. D. Dr. S. Wysocki, Chirurgische Universitätsklinik, D-6900 Heidelberg, Kirschnerstraße

Welcome

K. BARTMANN

My dear lady colleague and gentlemen!

It is really a great pleasure for me to welcome you to our symposium which is the third one. I thank you for accepting the invitation, especially those of you who have had a long journey.

The basic idea of these symposia is to give a small group of scientists the opportunity to deal with, and to discuss an important and current item of medicine in a quiet atmosphere with plenty of time. The first symposium was devoted to problems of immunology, the second to catechol amines.

Our subject, changes of causative agents in bacterial infections, is of interest from biological, epidemiological and therapeutic points of view. It implies problems of general biology, pathogenicity, host resistance and iatrogenic influences. We have tried to cover the subject as completely as possible. I thank very much Dr. FINLAND and Dr. MARGET for their great and continuous help in reaching this target. But it is quite clear from the programme as it looks now that we will miss some important aspects. This is in part due to the fact that some colleagues were unable to attend and had to cancel their participation in the last minute. Omissions are further due to lack of knowledge. For instance, this holds true for the present status of virulence. Except for a few bacterial species we dont' know their current virulence for experimental animals and moreover we don't know the meaning of virulence tests for human beings. But I hope that the discusion will fill the gaps to some extent.

The original meaning of the word symposium in Greek has nothing to do with science but much with enjoying life. I think, at least in the evening we should try to realize the original meaning to some extent, transformed into our present-day way of life, but still in the spirit of PLATON and of EPIKUR as well.

I. Bacterial Infections:
Changes in their Causative Agents. Trends

Bayer-Symposium III, 4—18 (1971)
© by Springer-Verlag 1971

Changing Prevalence of Pathogenic Bacteria in Relation to Time and the Introduction and Use of New Antimicrobial Agents*

M. FINLAND

It should be pointed out, at the very start, that the material to be presented under the title assigned to me is a sort of replay of an old record (FINLAND, 1970; FINLAND, JONES and BARNES, 1959), but in a new edition, with some different material to bring it more nearly up to date in line with some new developments. The bulk of the data consists primarily of surveys of material from the Boston City Hospital where we have been monitoring serious infections over the course of several decades. The first portion will deal with the bacteria which have been isolated from blood cultures of patients with compatible infections, and the changes in the frequency with which different bacterial pathogens have been encountered.

Background Data: Hospital Admissions

A few bits of background information will serve as sort of denominators for some of the data to be presented. First is the number of admissions to all services of the main general hospital each year over the period of the study; this has declined steadily from a peak of about 43,000 in 1941 to about 33,000 in 1961, and then the annual number of admissions stabilized at that figure through 1965. This represents about a 25% drop in the number of admissions to this hospital over the 25 years. Second, the number of deaths over the three decades between 1935 and 1965 declined more or less steadily from nearly 3,000 to just under 2,000 annually, a drop of about one-third for the entire period. Third, the mortality rate for all hospital admissions showed some fluctuations up to 1947, after which it dropped progressively from about 7.3% in that year to about 6% in 1965, a decline of about one-sixth over less than two decades.

Incidence and Mortality of All Bacteremic Infections

Data concerning all patients with bacteremia were collected for 10 selected years to reflect the impact of the introduction and widespread use of the successive antibacterial agents that became available over this interval. Only organisms considered to be true pathogens related to compatible infections in the patients were included. For the present purpose, organisms commonly found as contaminants (*Staphylococcus albus* and diphtheroids are examples) were totally excluded, even when repeatedly cultured, and when they clearly did cause disease.

* Most of the studies on which this paper is based were supported in part by grants 5R01-AI-00023 and 2T01-AI-00068 from the National Institute of Allergy and Infectious Disease.

The year 1935 was selected to represent the situation just before the sulfonamides were introduced; 1941 was chosen to reflect the effects of those agents just prior to the introduction of penicillin; 1947 to reflect the full impact of the use of penicillin and streptomycin before the first broadspectrum antibiotics, Aureomycin (chlortetracycline) and Chloromycetin (chloramphenicol), became available. The year 1951 was chosen as the year when penicillin-resistant staphylococci had become very common and before the first "anti-staphylococcal" antibiotic (erythromycin) was introduced, and 1961 was the year before the new semisynthetic penicillins and cephalosporins became available. Intervening years between 1951 and 1961 and additional years after that were also included to verify any trends.

In marked contrast to the steadily declining numbers of admissions to the hospital for all causes with the declining numbers of deaths and drop in mortality rate among those patients, there was a steady and marked increase in the annual number of bacteremic patients in the hospital and in the number of deaths among the bacteremic patients. Over the entire period of this study, the number of bacteremic patients increased steadily, from under 300 in 1935 to over 1,000 in 1965. The number of deaths in patients with verified bacteremic infections dropped slightly over the early years, just after the first introduction of effective antibacterial agents, from 168 in 1935 to 143 in 1947. The number of deaths in bacteremic patients then rose gradually but steadily to 400 in 1965. The case-fatality ratio, which was nearly 60% for all bacteremic patients in 1935, dropped sharply after the sulfonamides became widely used and dropped further to 30% in 1947 following the availability of penicillin and streptomycin. After the introduction of the broad-spectrum antibiotics the mortality rate among the bacteremic patients showed a steady increase to more than 40% in 1961, after which there was a slight tendency of the mortality to decline following the general availability of the semisynthetic penicillins and cephalosporins. However, the changes in case-fatality ratios varied with the different bacterial invaders, as will be detailed later.

Age has always been recognized as a major determining factor in the case-fatality ratio from various specific infections and this was equally true for the patients with bacteremia due to each of the various specific categories and for all the bacteremic patients combined. Beginning with a varying case-fatality ratio in those under 10 years old (most of those deaths being in newborns and in infants under 2 years old), the mortality dropped to its lowest rate in the second and third decades of life and then rose steeply for each advancing decade. The case-fatality ratio for patients in each decade of life during the 10 selected years reflected the overall decline for all ages through 1947, rising after that until 1961 and then declining again through 1965.

Factors Related to Changing Mortality: Age of the Patients

I shall not undertake to analyze all the factors entering into the changes in the overall mortality rates in bacteremic patients except as they relate to the changes in the age distribution of all the bacteremic patients over the period of this study. Table 1 shows the distribution of the bacteremic *patients* by decades of age for each of the 10 selected years of the study and Table 2 shows the corresponding data for the bacteremic *patients who died*. In Table 1 it is seen that in the years 1935 and 1941 the bacteremic patients were distributed more or less evenly over the various decades of age, especially between the ages of 10 and 69 years; there was a sharp drop in the numbers of patients of 70 years or older and there were none more than 90 years old. Beginning in 1947, the age distribution of the patients changed markedly, the proportion of those between 10 and 40 years old dropping steadily, while the proportion of those 70 years of age or older were increasing even more strikingly, and there were also appreciable, and increasing numbers of patients in the tenth decade of life.

Table 1. *Age distribution of patients with bacteremia, Boston City Hospital (ten selected years, 1935—1965)*

Year	Number of patients, age (years)										
	<10	10—19	20—29	30—39	40—49	50—59	60—69	70—79	80—89	90 +	Total
1935	23	34	53	38	40	43	39	18	3	0	291
1941	53	42	54	60	60	64	44	34	11	0	422
1947	30	37	52	58	57	74	75	67	18	1	469
1951	24	27	30	37	65	63	99	86	45	2	478
1953	39	21	41	59	51	74	110	113	61	2	571
1955	79	23	26	33	64	72	96	102	75	4	574
1957	124	15	25	23	49	65	100	112	79	6	598
1961	113	21	72	50	66	97	122	164	81	9	795
1963	110	21	48	68	97	137	132	177	100	20	910
1965	137	17	47	64	112	125	165	238	143	28	1076

Year	Distribution, percent of total, age (years)									
	<10	10—19	20—29	30—39	40—49	50—59	60—69	70—79	80—89	90 +
1935	7.9	11.7	18.2	13.1	13.7	14.8	13.4	6.2	1.0	0
1941	12.6	10.0	12.8	14.2	14.2	15.2	10.4	8.1	2.6	0
1947	6.4	7.9	11.1	12.4	12.2	15.8	16.0	14.3	3.8	0.2
1951	5.0	5.6	6.3	7.7	13.6	13.2	20.7	18.0	9.4	0.4
1953	6.8	3.7	7.2	10.3	8.9	13.0	19.3	19.8	10.7	0.4
1955	13.8	4.0	4.5	5.7	11.1	12.5	16.7	17.8	13.1	0.7
1957	20.7	2.5	4.2	3.8	8.2	10.9	16.7	18.7	13.2	1.0
1961	14.2	2.6	9.1	6.3	8.3	12.2	15.4	20.6	10.2	1.1
1963	12.1	2.3	5.3	7.5	10.6	15.1	14.5	19.5	11.5	2.2
1965	12.7	1.6	4.4	6.0	10.4	11.6	16.3	22.1	13.3	2.6

These changes in age distribution are even more striking among the bacteremic patients who died. Most noteworthy were first, the fact that for some of the years of the study, beginning in 1953, there were either no deaths at all, or only 1 or 2 deaths among bacteremic patients in the second and third decades of life; second, the numbers and proportions of those over 70 years of age rose steadily; and third, there were increasing numbers of patients and deaths among bacteremic patients 90 years of age or older. It is of particular interest to point out that there were *40% more bacteremic patients and 27% more deaths among those bacteremic patients over 70 years in the year 1965, as compared to the corresponding totals for all ages in the year 1935.*

Other Contributing Factors

Many factors other than age (though some were related to the advanced age of the patients) influenced the increased occurrence of bacteremic infections. The changes in the character of the bacterial invaders and in mortality was similar in many respects to those which are also generally related to nosocomial (hospital-acquired) infections, a large number of which are included among these cases. They also involve organisms formerly considered to be nonpathogenic, or at most mildly pathogenic—the so-called opportunistic pathogens. These contributing

Table 2. *Age distribution of deaths among patients with bacteremia, Boston City Hospital (ten selected years, 1935—1965)*

| Year | Number of deaths, age (years) | | | | | | | | | | Total |
	<10	10—19	20—29	30—39	40—49	50—59	60—69	70—79	80—89	90 +	
1935	7	7	18	27	25	32	32	17	3	0	168
1941	11	13	12	12	19	34	24	22	9	0	156
1947	9	2	2	9	14	33	31	35	7	1	143
1951	4	2	2	4	11	24	52	40	27	1	167
1953	6	0	1	12	7	25	49	60	40	1	201
1955	7	1	0	4	13	20	44	63	54	3	209
1957	10	1	2	5	13	26	58	61	53	5	234
1961	12	2	5	10	25	39	65	94	53	8	313
1963	22	1	3	10	34	49	73	90	65	14	361
1965	20	0	4	20	36	41	66	121	72	20	400

| Year | Distribution, percent of total, age (years) | | | | | | | | | |
	<10	10—19	20—29	30—39	40—49	50—59	60—69	70—79	80—89	90 +
1935	4.2	4.2	10.7	16.1	14.9	19.0	19.0	10.1	1.9	0
1941	7.1	8.3	7.7	7.7	12.2	21.8	15.4	14.1	5.8	0
1947	6.3	1.4	1.4	6.3	9.8	23.1	21.7	24.5	4.9	0.7
1951	2.4	1.2	1.2	2.4	6.6	14.4	31.1	24.0	16.2	0.6
1953	3.0	0	0.5	6.0	3.5	12.4	24.4	29.9	19.9	0.5
1955	3.3	0.5	0	1.9	6.2	9.6	21.1	30.1	25.8	1.4
1957	4.3	0.4	0.9	2.1	5.6	11.1	24.8	26.1	22.6	2.1
1961	3.8	0.6	1.6	3.2	8.0	12.5	20.8	30.0	16.9	2.6
1963	6.1	0.3	0.8	2.8	9.4	13.6	20.2	24.9	18.0	3.9
1965	5.0	0	1.0	5.0	9.0	10.3	16.5	30.3	18.0	5.0

factors included multiple chronic, disabling and degenerative diseases; malignant diseases and the so-called autoimmune or collagen diseases; prolonged therapy of these and other conditions with immunosuppressive and corticosteroid drugs; the use of large doses of antimicrobial agents—often multiple agents, given simultaneously—particularly over long periods; the increasing use of endoscopies, intubations, tracheostomy tubes, indwelling venous and urethral catheters; resort to long operations of increasing complexity involving much manipulation and instrumentation, and insertion of foreign substances, particularly in cardiac surgery and organ transplantations. All of these, and others, appear to predispose to infections, sometimes recurrent, with organisms which are increasingly resistant to more and more of the antimicrobial agents that are commonly used. Data on the role of these factors will not be presented here. I have recently reviewed the changing antibiotic resistance patterns among the bacteria encountered over the period of this study (FINLAND, 1971), so I shall not consider that aspect here.

Bacteremia Due to Specific Organisms

In addition to changes in age distribution of the patients with bacteremia the major changes that followed the introduction and widespread use of the succession of antibacterial agents was the altered incidence of the different etiologic bacteria causing the invasive infections. Notable has been the relative stability of the frequency with which certain bacteria have been found in bacteremic patients each year; outstanding in this respect have been the pneumococci and the viridans group (apha hemolytic, and gamma or nonhemolytic) of streptococci. Over the same period, the occurrence of other organisms, notably group A beta hemolytic streptococci declined sharply; still others fluctuated in incidence (*Staphylococcus aureus* being the most striking example), whereas the group of "enterobacteria", which includes the enterococci and the gram-negative bacilli—other than the usual enteric pathogens, namely Salmonella and Shigella—increased steadily in numbers and in relative incidence, and new species appeared and assumed importance as causes of serious bacteremic infections over the 35 year period of the study. It is therefore of some interest to summarize the changes in the numbers and relative incidence of cases and deaths among patients with bacteremia due to the more important of the specific bacterial species.

Diplococcus pneumoniae

Pneumococcal pneumonia was the most frequent of the serious conditions encountered on the medical wards of the Boston City Hospital during about half of each year when I first went there as an intern in 1927, and it remained so until well into the antibiotic era. Next to the advanced age of the patient, the demonstration of pneumococcal bacteremia was the most serious prognostic feature in the cases of pneumonia. In a study of the clinical significance of bacteremia in the cases of pneumococcal pneumonia observed at that hospital between November 1929 and May 1935 (TILGHMAN and FINLAND, 1937) the mortality rates in *all* cases were shown to rise steadily with increasing age—from 10% in the 10 to 19 years old to about 90% in those 70 years of age or older. The corresponding case-fatality ratios for the nonbacteremic patients ranged from about 7% to nearly 80%, whereas in those with positive blood cultures they ranged from 27% to 100%. Within each decade of age, except in the "70 and over" category, the case-fatality ratio was $2^1/_2$- to 6-fold greater in bacteremic than in nonbacteremic patients. The proportion of patients with pneumonia in which bacteremia was demonstrated also rose steadily with advancing age, from 15% in those 10 to 19 years old to nearly 60% in the seventh decade of life, but it was slightly lower in those over 70 years old.

The present study includes patients with pneumococcal bacteremia from all causes (pneumonia, meningitis, peritonitis, and "cryptogenic" cases or those without demonstrable foci) and, although pneumonia accounted for the great majority of the cases, the deaths included a large proportion of others, notably those with meningitis. Over the 30 years of the study there were moderate fluctuations in the numbers of patients with pneumococcal bacteremia seen during each of the 10 selected years, but the average and median numbers were about 100 cases annually.

In 1935, pneumococcal bacteremia accounted for slightly more than one-third of all bacteremic patients observed in the hospital and nearly one-half of all the deaths in patients with bacteremic infections, and the case-fatality ratio among these bacteremic pneumococcal infections was 78%. Following the successive introduction of effective sulfonamide drugs and penicillin, the proportion of all bacteremic infections that were due to pneumococci dropped to 21%; that of the deaths in these bacteremic cases dropped to 18% and the case-fatality ratio dropped first to 36% under the impact of the sulfonamides, and then to 21% after penicillin came into use. After 1947, the proportion of the bacteremic patients due to *Pneumococcus* stabilized at about 14% of all bacteremic patients and at about 10% of the deaths among those patients, with the case-fatality ratio in the patients with pneumococcal bacteremia hovering around 25%.

Beta-Hemolytic Streptococci (Group A)

The organism which ranked second in importance, from the point of view of mortality, among bacteremic patients, was the beta-hemolytic streptococcus. In the earlier years some of the strains were presumed and others proved to be group A, whereas during most of the study nearly all were definitely identified as group A. KEEFER, INGELFINGER and SPINK (1937) analyzed 246 cases of beta hemolytic streptococcal bacteremia that occurred at Boston City Hospital, all but a few of them before the introduction of sulfonamides. The mortality in all these cases was more than 70%. The incidence of bacteremia, and the case-fatality ratio in those cases rose steadily with increasing age of the patients.

In 1935, the first year of the present study, beta hemolytic streptococcus was the causative organism in 18% of all bacteremic infections and nearly one-fourth of all deaths from such infections at this hospital. These proportions dropped sharply after the introduction and use of the sulfonamide drugs to 4% of all bacteremic cases and 7% of the deaths in 1941. After that, the decline continued until 1955 when group A beta hemolytic streptococcus accounted for less than 1% of all bacteremic infections and there were *no deaths* due to this organism in that year. Subsequently the number of patients and deaths has been rising steadily until 1965, when 4.4% of all bacteremic patients and 5% of deaths from all invasive infections were due to this organism. The case-fatality ratio since 1961 has ranged from 31% to 45%, the large majority of the fatal cases being recognized late in the disease or as a terminal event in serious chronic diseases.

Staphylococcus aureus

Ranking third among the causative organism of serious bacteremic infections at the start of this study was *Staphylococcus aureus*. An analysis of 122 cases of bacteremia due to *Staphylococcus aureus* which occurred at this hospital between 1934 and 1941 was published by SKINNER and KEEFER (1941). The mortality in those cases was 82% and nearly all of the survivors were under 40 years old. The largest number of patients were in the second decade of age; the incidence declined, but the case-fatality increased with advancing age.

In 1935, the first year of the present study, *Staphylococcus aureus* accounted for 22% of all bacteremic patients and 18% of all deaths among such patients. There was an epidemic of staphylococcal pneumonia complicating influenca A in 1941, when there were 145 patients and 43 deaths due to bacteremic staphylococcal infections. Excluding that year, there was a steady increase in the number of patients with staphylococcal bacteremia from 66 in 1935 to 225 in 1957; after that the number dropped appreciably, but there were still 192 cases in 1965. The proportion of all patients with bacteremic infections that were caused by *Staph. aureus* rose to nearly 40% in 1955 and 1957, and the same was true of the proportion of deaths among all bacteremic infections; these proportions dropped back to 18% and 19% respectively by 1965. The case-fatality ratio among the patients with bacteremia due to *Staph. aureus* dropped from 47% in 1935 to 30% in 1941 and to 19% in 1947, but after that year it rose steadily to 48% in 1961 and then dropped again to 35% in 1956.

Viridans Streptococci

The number of patients with bacteremia due to *Streptococcus viridans*, in which are included both the alpha hemolytic and the gamma streptococci, varied only moderately and irregularly in the different years of the stufy, around a mean and median of 49 patients for the 10 selected years. The pathogenic significance of these organisms is often in question, except in well-defined clinical cases of subacute bacterial endocarditis, because these are common as transient invaders of the blood stream, generally from the mouth, in patients with poor dental hygiene and periodental infections. Although patients with proved endocarditis were included, they constituted a minority each year, but all of the patients who were included had positive blood cultures for these organisms on repeated occasions, were febrile, or had some other focal lesion such as meningitis, pneumonia or empyema from which the same organism and no other significant pathogen was recovered. Some of those patient may have been in an early stage of *endocarditis lenta* which was lacking the classical peripheral signs and which, in those who recovered, may have responded favorably to therapy with effective antibiotics—usually penicillin, alone or with streptomycin, and thus that diagnosis could not be fully confirmed.

In 1935, the patients with bacteremia due to *Streptococcus viridans* constituted about 15% of all the bacteremia patients and 12% of the cases that were fatal. This proportion declined steadily until 1953 to 6% of all bacteremic patients and about 3% of the cases that were fatal, and remained at that level with some aberrations in 1 or 2 of the subsequent years of the study. The case-fatality ratio in these cases was 48%, in 1935, dropped in successive stages to 11% by 1951, but varied irregularly between 13% and 27% after that year.

Enterococcus (Group D Streptococcus)

Enterococcus, generally identified also as group D streptococci, and which included mostly *Streptococcus zymogenes*, *Str. liquefaciens*, *Str. faecalis* and its subspecies and a few *Str. faecium*, appears to be one of the new group of organisms that have emerged during the antibiotic era, at least as a cause of bacteremic infections, including bacterial endocarditis. In 1935 there were *no* cases at all in which such organisms were identified from blood cultures as a pathogen. Four cases were recognized in 1941, but since then the number has increased irregularly to 61 patients in 1965; they constituted 1% of all bacteremic patients and 1.3% of deaths in such cases in 1941, increasing to 6.1% and 6.7%, respectively in 1965. The case-fatality ratio was 50% or more from 1941 through 1951, then dropped to about 30% by 1957 but subsequently increased again to nearly 50%. Bacteremias due to these organisms have their origin most frequently in infections of the urinary tract.

Gram-Negative Bacilli

The most striking and persistent change in the causative organisms in patients with bacteremic infections since effective antibacterial agents have come into wide use, has been the steady increase in the numbers and proportions of patients in whom the bacteremic infections were due to gram-negative bacilli. In this category of bacteria, sometimes referred to in clinical reports as "gram-negative rods", are included "enteric" organisms (coliforms, Proteus, Pseudomonas, Herellea, Mima, Klebsiella, etc.) other than the usual "enteric pathogens" such as Salmonella and Shigella. Most of these organisms have usually been associated with the normal fecal flora and were not generally considered to be highly pathogenic. This group of organisms is, for convenience, called "enterobacteria"—and the enterococci have been included under this term. I shall limit the presentation to some of the species of the gram-negative bacilli of this group which have been occurring in increasing numbers over most of the period of the present study, with brief reference to certain other species which have newly emerged more recently and involved rather large numbers of patients.

Escherichia coli

The most common of the gram-negative enterobacteria causing bacteremic infections at the Boston City Hospital is *Escherichia coli*. This is the only one of the group that caused appreciable numbers of cases of bacteremic infections prior to the introduction of the sulfonamide drugs. In 1935, the first year of the present study, about 9% of all bacteremic patients and 6% of the deaths among such patients were due to this organism. From 27 cases in 1935, the number increased to 46 and 70 in 1941 and 1947, respectively, corresponding to 11% and 15% of all bacteremic infections and deaths from such infections, respectively. There were about 60 such infections, representing 9 to 12% of all bacteremic patients in each of the next selected years of the study (to 1961) after which the number increased sharply to 114 patients in 1963 and 140 in 1965, corresponding to 13% and 14% of all patients with bacteremic infections in those years.

The case-fatality ratios in the patients with bacteremia due to *E. coli* fluctuated irregularly within the range between 36% and 49% over the 30 years of the study and these patients accounted for 10 to 14% of all the deaths from bacteremic infections in the years selected for this study. Interestingly enough, the case-fatality ratios in the first 4 selected years (1935 to 1951) ranged from 36 to 39%

and it was 36% in 1965, but in all but one of the 5 intervening years that were studied (1953 to 1963) the case-fatality tanged between 43 and 49%. During the entire period of the study, by far the most frequent source of *E. coli* in the bacteremic patients has been infection of the urinary tract, but infections of the respiratory tract due to this organism are being recognized with increasing frequency in recent years.

Proteus Species

Organisms of the genus *Proteus* had been encountered as a cause of bacteremic infections prior to the antibiotic era, but they were infrequent. There were 6 such cases of infections with 5 deaths at Boston City Hospital in 1935, and 7 cases with 3 deaths in 1941. In the other 8 selected years, from 1947 through 1965, the number of patients with bacteremia due to *Proteus* varied irregularly between 25 and 65 (mean 48, median 49), but the case-fatality ratio, which reached a low of 28% in 1951, increased more or less progressively thereafter to 69% in 1963, and it was 58% in 1965. The proportion of all patients with bacteremic infections that were due to *Proteus* rose from about 2% in 1935 and 1941 to a peak of 13% in 1951, and then declined more or less steadily to 4% and 5% in the last 2 selected years of the study. Among all the fatal bacteremic infections, *Proteus* accounted for increasing proportions—from 2% to 17%—between 1941 and 1955 and the proportion declined to between 6% and 8% from 1961 through 1965. The great majority of the strains of *Proteus* at this hospital have been identified biochemically as *P. mirabilis* on occassions when they were specifically studied for other purposes (ADLER et al., 1971; FRANK et al., 1950; POTEE et al., 1954)—72% in 1954 (POTEE et al., 1954) and 87% in 1970 (ADLER et al., 1971) of *all* proteus infections (not just bacteremias) being classified as *P. mirabilis*.

Pseudomonas aeruginosa

Another of the gram-negative bacilli that were rarely encountered as a cause of invasive infection before the modern era of chemotherapy and which have come into prominence in the period of this study is *Pseudomonas aeruginosa*. This organism was responsible for only a single bacteremic infection in 1935, for 5 cases of such infections in 1941 and 8 in 1947. In each of the succeeding 5 selected years, 1951 through 1961, there were between 14 and 20 (mean 17) patients with bacteremia due to *Pseudomonas*, but in 1963 and 1965 there were 48 and 50 such patients, respectively. These infections accounted for 3 to 4% of all cases of bacteremic infection at this hospital during most of the years of the study and for 7 and 9% during the last 2 years. The overall case-fatality ratio in all the cases in the 10 selected years was 55%, but in different years it ranged from a low of 40% in 1961 to a high of 66% in 1965, the median being 60%.

Klebsiella-Enterobacter (Aerobacter)

In the recent taxonomy and nomenclature (EWING, 1966) used in the United States, as recommended by the National Communicable Disease Center (now known as the Center for Disease Control), one of the principal divisions of the family *Enterobacteriaceae* is the tribe Klebsielleae. This tribe consists of three genera: *Klebsiella, Enterobacter* (formerly called *Aerobacter*) and *Serratia*. In our clinical experience, the only species that are important as causes of serious infections within this division are *K. pneumoniae, E. aerogenes, E. cloacae* and *S. marcescens;* most strains of the last species that have been isolated in recent years have been nonpigmented. There are now 72 specific capsular serotypes of *K. pneumoniae,* of which types 1 and 2, formerly designated *Friedländer's bacillus* types A and B, had been recognized as not infrequent causes of infections of the respiratory and urinary tracts at Boston City Hospital prior to the advent of the sulfonamide drugs. Antisera for serotypes 3, 4 and 5 (*Friedländer's bacillus* types C, D and E) were also available, but strains of these types were only rarely encountered. Strains of *K. pneumoniae* of types other than 1 to 5, and strains of *Enterobacter* of both species began to appear, or at least to be recognized, as causes of serious infections only after penicillin and streptomycin had come into wide use. Infections due to *Serratia* have come into prominence only since 1961 and reports dealing with *S. marcescens* and infections associated with it have been published recently from our hospital (WILFERT et al., 1970; WILFERT et al., 1968).

In order to emphasize the changing pattern of infections during the antibiotic era, I have segregated the strains of *K. pneumoniae,* other than those of types 1 to 5, and those of *Enterobacter* of both species and shall consider the three species together under the designation Klebsiella—Enterobacter which, as "Klebsiella—Aerobacter", has been widely referred to by clinical bacteriologists and in many reports in the literature. There were *no* cases of bacteremic infections due to Klebsiella—Enterobacter (as defined here) recognized at Boston City Hospital during the first 2 selected years of this study—1935 and 1941—that is, prior to the availability of penicillin and streptomycin. In 1947, after those two antibiotics and the effective sulfonamides had achieved wide use, there were 46 cases with 20 deaths, and in 1951—after tetracycline, chloramphenicol and polymyxin B had come into general use—there were 41 patients with bacteremic infections due to Klebsiella—Enterobacter of whom 15 died; the case-fatality ratios in these 2 years being 44% and 57%, respectively.

During the next 4 selected years of the study, the number of cases of bacteremic infections due to Klebsiella—Enterobacter ranged from 45 to 58, and the number of deaths in those cases ranged from 25 to 31, the case-fatality ratios for the different years being 50 to 59%. In the last 2 of the selected years of the study —1963 and 1965—the number of patients with these infections increased to 71 and 80, and the case-fatality for those years was 59 and 43%, respectively. From 1947 through 1965, the proportion of all bacteremic patients in this hospital that were due to Klebsiella—Enterobacter varied from 8 to 10%, and they accounted for 10 to 16% of all deaths due to bacteremic infection.

"Enterobacteria"

In order to bring into still sharper focus the important role of the new species of organisms that has emerged, I have grouped together under the term "enterobacteria" the enterococci, all of the species of gram-negative bacilli that were already discussed in some detail in the preceding sections, and in addition, such "new" infections as those due to *Serratia, Mima,* and *Herellea,* which have assumed particular prominence during the last years of the study, but excluding *Salmonella, Shigella* and certain others to be mentioned later in a "miscellaneous" category. None of the "miscellaneous" species showed any appreciable change in numbers during the years of this study. In the year 1965 alone there were 58 patients with bacteremia due to *Herellea vaginicola*, of whom 21 died; 27 patients and 6 deaths due to *Mima polymorpha*, and 12 cases with 5 deaths in patients with bacteremia due to *S. marcescens*. When considered together, these "enterobacteria" accounted for a steadily and markedly increasing number and proportion of the bacteremic patients and deaths in this hospital during the antibiotic era.

In 1935, there were 34 cases and 15 deaths in patients with bacteremia due to such enterobacteria, nearly all of them due to *E. coli* or *Proteus* species. These numbers were nearly doubled in 1941, and increased again nearly three-fold from those numbers by 1947, when there were 176 such patients with 69 deaths. The increase continued steadily, but was less precipitate over the next 5 selected years, so that by 1961 there were 260 cases with 126 deaths among patients with bacteremia due to enterobacteria. There was then a further and accelerate increase to 389 patients and 188 deaths in 1963, and to 480 patients with 197 deaths in 1965. The case-fatality ratios over the entire period of study ranged from a low of 35% in 1951 to a high of 53% in 1957, and dropping back to 41% in 1965, the mean and median for all the cases in the 10 selected years being 44%. The proportion of all bacteremic patients in each of the 10 selected years that were due to enterobacterial infections ranged from 12% in 1935 to 48% in 1965, and the corresponding proportion of the deaths in those years ranged from 9% in 1935 to a high of 58% in 1955, and it was 55% in 1965.

Miscellaneous Infections

If we now consider together all of the remaining patients with bacteremic infections not discussed in the preceding sections, we have a miscellaneous group, which includes streptococci of serological groups other than A and D, *Hemophilus influenzae*, *Neisseria (meningitidis* and *gonorrhoeae)*, *Salmonella*, clostridia, and others were encountered in small numbers. These miscellaneous infections together constituted a slightly decreasing proportion of cases and deaths among bacteremic patients over the years of this study, from 20% of all patients and 15% of all deaths in 1935 to 15% of the cases and 9% of deaths in 1965, and some still lower figures in the intervening years.

As already noted, I excluded all patients in whom the only organisms cultured from blood, even on repeated occassions, were *Staphylococcus albus (S. epidermidis)*, *Bacillus subtilis*, diphtheroids or others commonly considered to be contaminants, even if they were clearly causing infection. In an earlier report (Finland, Jones and Barnes, 1959), an attempt was made to evaluate the contribution of *S. albus* to the problem of bacteremia. The number of patients who had *S. albus* in more than one blood culture, and the case-fatality ratio in those patients were more or less constant between 1935 and 1957 (inclusive). The role of this species in bacterial endocarditis during the years of this study was discussed recently (Finland and Barnes, 1970).

Summary and Comment

The changes in the causative organisms of bacteremic infections observed at Boston City Hospital fall into four categories:

1. The first category includes organisms which were the major cause of bacteremic infections, and of mortality from such infections before the era of modern antibacterial therapy, and which declined markedly in relation to the total numbers of cases and particularly as a cause of death due to bacteremic infections, after the effective antibacterial agents came into wide use. They include primarily *the pneumococci and the group A beta hemolytic streptococci* which, together, *accounted for one-half of all bacteremic infections and nearly two-thirds of all deaths from such infections in 1935.* Following the introduction and use of sulfonamides and penicillin, these ratios declined promptly, and since then these organisms have been responsible for about 1 of every 6 patients with bacteremia and for 1 in 7 to 10 of all deaths among bacteremic patients. Of some concern, however, has been the resurgence of group A beta hemolytic streptococci since 1961.

2. The second category, at the opposite extreme, includes the group of organisms that were lumped together under the designation "enterobacteria"; the number of bacteremic patients with infections due to these organisms, and of deaths among such patients, has increased steadily throughout the years of this study, with new species appearing and gaining some prominence.

3. The third category includes bacteremic infections caused by a wide variety of common pathogenic organisms which have been occurring regularly in small or moderate numbers throughout the years of this study; the most frequent of these were the viridans streptococci, but also including hemolytic streptococci other than those of group A, anaerobic and microaerophilic streptococci, *Neisseria*, clostridia, *H. influenzae, Salmonella, Shigella* as well as a host of others which were lumped together as "miscellaneous" organisms.

4. The fourth category includes only infections with *Staphylococcus aureus* which increased steadily through 1957, then leveled off in 1961 and finally showed a tendency to decline in number and in their proportions relative to all the patients with bacteremic infections and to the deaths among such patients.

It is of interest that the steady or declining incidence and fatality, in categories 1 and 3, has been associated with organisms that are the most sensitive to available antibiotics, and which have retained that susceptibility, essentially without change. Increasing incidence and fatality, as in group 2, and in the group 4 (up to 1957), has been clearly associated with high degrees of resistance to antibiotics, either "innate" or acquired, and were fundamentally related to selection and spread of antibiotic-resistant organisms or variants under the impact and selective pressure of the intensive use of antibacterial agents for therapy, and particularly for prophylaxis. This aspect, insofar as it concerns material studied over the same period at Boston City Hospital, was reviewed at the *Conference on Problems of Drug Resistant Pathogenic Bacteria* sponsored by the New York Academy of Science just prior to the present Symposium and will be published in the report of that conference (FINLAND, 1971). I shall, therefore, not dwell further on this aspect, except as may be called for in relation to discussions of some of the other papers to be presented at this conference.

Of some concern, however, has been the recent reappearance and increase of bacteremic infections due to group A hemolytic streptococci, in spite of the fact that these organisms have retained their high degree of susceptibility to penicillin and to many other available antibiotics, although a moderate proportion of them have recently been found resistant to the tetracycline antibiotics (EICKHOFF and FINLAND, 1965; STEIGBIGEL et al., 1968). This is particularly disturbing because of the high case-fatality ratio among the recent cases of bacteremic infections due to the group A beta hemolytic streptococci. On the other hand, these recent cases have occurred predominantly among the aged, the infirm, those having one or more serious chronic diseases or malignat disease, those admitted in a neglected condition, and often as terminal events and even unrecognized, in patients dying of other conditions. They also include some patients on treatment with immuno-suppressive agents, and others in whom the first evidence of the streptococcal infection was the result of a premortem or even post-mortem culture.

Mention has already been made of the possible role played in the rising incidence of bacteremic infections by the increasing use of new, long and complicated operations by greater resort to tracheal intubations, tracheostomies, endoscopies, indwelling catheters in blood vessels and various body orifies, by the long-term use of many drugs, particularly antitumor agents, immunosuppressives, and corticosteroids, and by the insertion of foreign bodies such as valves and trans-plants and by the use of excessive doses and numbers of antimicrobial agents, —many of them gratuitously. The role of these factors has been noted but not specifically evaluated. However, the effect of the marked increase in age of patients with bacteremia has been clearly documented as a major contributor to the increased incidence and mortality of all the bacteremic infections.

The changes in the relative incidence and mortality of infections due to *Staphylococcus aureus*, have been related to the appearance and increase first of penicillin-resistant (penicillinase producing) strains (FINLAND and HAIGHT, 1953), then of the appearance and increase of staphylococci of certain specific phage patterns—notably 52/42B/81 during the early 1950's (FINLAND, JONES and BARNES, 1959), followed by those of the 80/81 group (WALLMARK and FINLAND, 1961) and finally a decrease in predominance of the 80/81 strains (BARRETT et al., 1970). These changes were accompanied by changes in hospital from a predomi-nance of group III to that of group I and then a tendency to a return of the group III phages, with the reverse being true of staphylococci isolated in the community (BARRETT et al., 1970; WALLMARK and FINLAND, 1961).

That many or most of the changes described here are not limited to the Boston City Hospital or similar institutions, but have also occurred to varying degrees elsewhere has been well documented from many hospitals in advanced countries throughout the world, but I shall not review these reports here. However, it should be noted that similar changes in bacterial ecology of invasive infections have been reported in children (SHALLARD and WILLIAMS, 1965), especially in newborns (KLEIN, 1969) and also in obstetrical patients, particularly in septic abortions (SMITH et al., 1970; WEINGOLD et al., 1966).

Perhaps the clearest reflection of the changes in the occurrence and nature of bacteremic infections is seen in the changes in the etiology of well-documented cases of bacterial endocarditis during the same years of the study. These cases have been reported elsewhere (FINLAND and BARNES, 1970).

References

ADLER, J. L., BURKE, J. P., WILCOX, C., FINLAND, M.: Susceptibility of *Preoteus species* and *Pseudomonas aeruginosa* to penicillins and cephalosporins. Antimicrobial Agents & Chemother. — 1970, 63—67 (1971).

BARRETT, F. F., CASEY, J. I., WILCOX, C., FINLAND, M.: Bacteriophage types and antibiotic susceptibility of *Staphylococcus aureus:* Boston City Hospital, 1967. Arch. Intern. Med. 125, 867—873 (1970).

EICKHOFF, T. C., FINLAND, M.: *In vitro* susceptibility of group A beta hemolytic streptococci to 18 antibiotics. Amer. J. med. Sci. 249, 261—268 (1965).

EWING, W. H.: Enterobacteriaceae, taxonomy and nomenclature. U.S. Dept. Health, Education and Welfare, Public Health Service, Bureau of Disease Prevention and Environmental Control, National Communicable Disease Center, Atlanta, Georgia, December 1966, 23 pages.

FINLAND, M.: Changing ecology of bacterial infections as related to antibacterial therapy. J. infect. Dis. 122, 419—431 (1970).

— Changes in susceptibility of selected pathogenic bacteria to widely used antibiotics (presented at a Conference on the Problems of Drug Resistant Pathogenic Bacteria sponsored by the New York Academy of Sciences, October 12, 1970). Ann. N.Y. Acad. Sci. 182, 5—20 (1971).

— BARNES, M. W.: Changing etiology of bacterial endocarditis in the antibacterial era. Experiences at Boston City Hospital 1933—1965. Ann. intern. Med. 72, 341—348 (1970).

— HAIGHT, T. H.: Antibiotic resistance of pathogenic staphylococci: Study of five hundred strains isolated at Boston City Hospital from October 1951 to February 1952. Arch. intern. Med. 91, 143—158 (1953).

— JONES, W. F., Jr., BARNES, M. W.: Occurrence of serious infections since the introduction of antibacterial agents. J. Amer. med. Ass. 170, 2188—2197 (1959).

— — BENNETT, I. L., Jr.: Antibiotic susceptibility and phage types of pathogenic staphylococci. A study of two hundred ten strains isolated at Boston City Hospital in 1955. Arch. intern. Med. 104, 365—377 (1959).

FRANK, P. F., WILCOX, C., FINLAND, M.: *In vitro* sensitivity of *Bacillus proteus* and *Pseudomonas* to seven antibiotics (penicillin, streptomycin, bacitracin, polymyxin, Aerosporin, Aureomycin and Chloromycetin). J. Lab. clin. Med. 35, 205—214 (1950).

KEEFER, C. S., INGELFINGER, F. J., SPINK, W. W.: Significance of hemolytic streptococcic bacteremia: a study of 246 patients. Arch. intern. Med. 60, 1084—1097 (1937).

KLEIN, J. O.: Considerations of gentamicin for therapy of neonatal sepsis. J. infect. Dis 119, 457—459 (1969).

POTEE, K. G., WRIGHT, S. S., FINLAND, M.: *In vitro* susceptibility of recently isolated strains of Proteus to ten antibiotics. J. Lab. clin. Med. 44, 463—477 (1954).

SHALLARD, M. A., WILLIAMS, A. L.: A study of the carriage of gram-negative bacilli by newborn babies in hospital. Med. J. Aust. 1, 504—542 (1965).

SKINNER, D., KEEFER, C. S.: Significance of bacteremia caused by *Staphylococcus aureus:* study of 122 cases and review of literature concerned with experimental infections in animals. Arch. intern. Med. 68, 851—875 (1941).

SMITH, J. W., SOUTHERN, P. M., Jr., LEHMANN, J. D.: Bacteremia in septic abortion: complications and treatment. Obstet gynec. Surv. 35, 704—708 (1970).

STEIGBIGEL, N. H., REED, C. W., FINLAND, M.: Susceptibility of common pathogenic bacteria to seven tetracycline antibiotics *in vitro*. Amer. J. med. Sci. 255, 179—195 (1968).

TILGHMAN, R. C., FINLAND, M.: Clinical significance of bacteremia in pneumococcal pneumonia. Arch. intern. Med. 59, 602—619 (1937).

WALLMARK, G., FINLAND, M.: Phage types and antibiotic susceptibility of pathogenic staphylococci. Results at Boston City Hospital 1959—1960 and comparison with strains of previous years. J. Amer. med. Sci. 175, 886—897 (1961).

Weingold, A. B., Gordon, M., Sall, J., Derry, J.: Bacteriologic studies of septic abortion. Pacif. Med. Surg. **76**, 8—9 (1966).
Wilfert, J.N., Barrett, F. F., Ewing,W. H., Finland, M., Kass, E. H.: *Serratia marcescens:* Biochemical, serological, and epidemiological characteristics and antibiotic susceptibility of strains isolated at Boston City Hospital. Appl. Microbiol. **19**, 345—352 (1970).
— — Kass, E. H.: Bacteremia due to *Serratia marcescens*. New Engl. J. Med. **279**, 286—289 (1968).

Prof. M. Finland
Department of Health and Hospitals
Channing Laboratory
Boston City Hospital
774 Albany Street
Boston, MA 02118, U.S.A.

Discussion

Gould: As always one is extremely impressed by Prof. Finland's figures for the increase in the incidence of bacteremia in Boston, particularly as caused by the gram-negative bacteria. I would like to ask first, what proportion of these patients does he think actually contracted the infection with these organisms, particularly the antibiotic resistant gram-negative bacteria, from the hospital environment? One reason I ask this is because I am particularly interested in the vast difference there is in the incidence he reports as compared with our own experience in Edinburgh. After a rapid calculation I find that the comparative figures for a general hospital in Edinburgh are 50 cases of bacteremia among 15,000 annual admissions, or approximately one tenth the rate reported from Boston, where there are 1,000 among 30,000 yearly admissions. Now do you think this is due to a difference in the use of antibiotics? Is there very much more being used or is it being used in a different way? It would appear to me that no matter how the techniques for demonstrating bacteremia should vary, there seems to be some fundamental reason for such a marked difference between the two places.

Finland: There are probably differences in the type of population that you deal with in different hospitals. I think our population, during this period, has been increasingly changed—with respect to age for one thing.

1. I have already mentioned the marked difference in the age distribution of the bacteremic patients from 1935 to 1965;—in the latter year there were 40% more patients with bacteremia over 70 years of age than there were total bacteremic patients in all age groups in 1935.

2. We are a public hospital that accepts all patients and we are required to accept the residue of patients after they have been discarded by other hospitals in the community, so that a large proportion of these patients that I mention are not only in the older age groups but they already have been in and out of hospitals and many of them bounce back and forth from nursing homes. Parenthetically a "Nursing Home" in the U.S.A. is different from a "Nursing Home" as you call it in Britain. As I understand it the "Nursing Home" in Britain is a private hospital whereas as "Nursing Home" in the United States is a place where you send the patients after you have nothing more to offer them in the hospital; it

serves as a repository until the patient again comes to a point where he requires more intensive therapy than is available in the nursing home and he is then returned to the hospital.

3. There has also been an increase in the number of gram-negative bacterial infections coming into our hospitals from the community (including the nursing homes). Most of that change has been in patients with urinary tract infections but we are also getting an increasing number of primary infections of the respiratory tract with gram-negative bacteria.

Dr. A. Martin Lerner and Dr. James R. Tillotson, working in Detroit, have been able to document the occurrence of primary gram-negative bacillary pneumonia in that community. Dr. Tillotson then spent a couple of years with us at Boston City Hospital and showed the same thing—an increasing number of patients with gram-negative pulmonary infections. But I think with respect to the hospital origin of these gram-negative bacterial infections, there is no doubt that a large proportion of them are nosocomial in origin. They occur in patients who come into the hospital either for primary pulmonary infections due to gram-positive organisms—shall we say pneumococcal pneumonia, and being of the older age group and debilitated, they often develop superinfections. First they are colonized with gram-negative bacteria and some get acute infection with these organisms. Some also develop bacteremia with a fatal outcome. Some of them come into the hospital for other reasons, usually with serious diseases and in bad general condition. They may have been alimented by vein or they have to be treated parenterally for other reasons and may develop infections by the venous route, or they have to be catheterized with urinary catheters after which some of them develop a hospital type of infection—secondary infections of the urinary tract. Thus there is no doubt that a large proportion of these strains are hospital-acquired and related, to some extent, to the character of the population and the type of therapy to which they are necessarily subjected.

Now I have not fully documented all of the background for these infections, there is no doubt that many of them are patients who have serious underlying diseases for which they receive various therapies. Many of them are patients who are admitted with paralytic central nervous system diseases or with cancerous diseases, for which they receive immunosuppressive agents and they develop these bacteremic infections while in the hospital. All of these factors enter into the large numbers and great increase in numbers of gram-negative bacteremias which we have seen here in recent years.

Kass: Perhaps other possibilities should be considered. I have looked at the comparative customs of hospitals in different countries. I do not know how important a variable it is, but the frequency with which cultures are taken is quite different in different places. For example, at the Boston City Hospital, about 150,000 cultures are taken annually. Approximately 100,000 of them are from in-patients and the remainder are from out-patients and from the community cultures. The 100,000 cultures are taken from about 27,000 patients admitted, or an average of close to four cultures per patient. Dr. Finland has taught us what he and we have all learned very quickly, that when a patient was about to receive an antibiotic and when it was necessary to change from one antibiotic to another, the minimum necessity was a blood culture and a culture of whatever other area

2*

looked relevant to the patient's problem. This was also true when the patient had a relapse of fever or was not otherwise responding to therapy. As a consequence, we found many patients who have positive blood cultures under circumstances in which they have low grade fevers, or other conditions that might not ordinarily have been considered, as a basis for taking cultures of the blood. This may be one of the variables that account for some of the differences in the data.

GOULD: The hospital customs are remarkably similar in Edinburgh with 55,000 specimens from the 15,000 admissions. How many blood cultures are taken in the Boston City Hospital each year?

FINLAND: I have considered this question in some detail. In the first year of our study (i.e. in 1935) there were 10,000 cultures done in all, including blood cultures. In the last year of the study (1965) there were over 110,000 and Dr. KASS mentioned that in most recent years it has reached over 150,000. It had been a sort of progressive increase, except for a brief period when very few blood cultures were taken in our paediatrics department. I think it is fair to say that no patient with a serious infection escaped having blood cultures done throughout the entire period of the study, the major difference being that in the earlier period, when a patient had bacteremia, he might have had one or two cultures and probably was not recultured many times after that. In the more recent period, since the introduction of the antimicrobial agents as Dr. KASS as indicated, we have tended to repeat cultures in all patients in whom either the fever persisted or recurred, in order to use it as a guide for our therapy. Moreover, more cultures were taken —multiple cultures were taken much more frequently in the recent years. There are two reasons for this—one is the interest in infections, and the other is the fact that there has been an increasing "academization", one might say, of our hospital. At the earlier part of this period Harvard was the one major academic unit and Tufts was beginning to demonstrate increasing academic interest but there was always teaching of Tufts students on both the medical and surgical wards. Boston University has also come in about the time when this study began and they have also increased their use of the bacteriology laboratory. In the last 20 years the paediatrics department has also become an academic service in which patients are treated and studied more intensively, so we had a large increase of culturing done on that service. These are some of the factors which have resulted in the large increase in the numbers of cultures. But as I have mentioned before, in going over records I do not think I have ever been able to determine a good base-line—it would take too much trouble—but I have come away with the feeling that there have been no patients, or rarely any, with serious infections, such as are included in these bacteremia studies, who have not had some culturing done.

WILLIAMS: Do the numbers of bacteremias represent cultures or patients?

FINLAND: I am glad you asked. Each number represents one patient but one patient and one organism—so that when we have a patient who comes in with a pneumococcemia and he recovers so that no pneumococci are found and then he has a staphylococcus, he would be included as a pneumococcus and as a staphylococcus bacteremia (that is, as two patients).

WILLIAMS: May I ask a more difficult question—I wonder whether you have had an opportunity of comparing the frequency of different bacteria in a more or less standard group of patients admitted at different periods of the survey ? As you said so many times during your presentation—there have been enormous changes in age distribution over the years and it is very difficult to extract, from the figures that we have, the therapeutic effects or the incidence of infections and on the nature of the infecting organisms; the changes in age of the patients, the changes in the prevalent diseases in the medical management and in the antibiotic management.

FINLAND: For some organisms unfortunately we have not had the opportunity to study all of these aspects over the years. However, we have some breakdown of the pneumococcal infections by age and pneumococcal bacteremias. The age distribution and the mortality has changed so that in the earlier period, that is in the 1930's before sulfonamides and before penicillin, we had an increase of 10% in the mortality for every succeeding decade of age. In more recent years, except in the first year or two of life, there is a constant and low mortality, until you get to the age of 50 or 60 and then it rises sharply. Unfortunately, we have not had an opportunity to study many of these cases but I have tried to indicate that we have done this recently for some of these cases. For example, in Dr. TILLOTSON's study, he recently followed a group of patients who came into the hospital with primary pneumonia to determine the changes that occur in the microbiology of the respiratory tract. During their stay in the hospital, he demonstrated a high rate of colonization with staphylococci and gram-negative bacteria, with a relatively modest increase in actual infection, that is, clinical infection, with these newly colonized organisms.

Now that's the sort of thing that I am sure should be done and which would give a clearer basis for the changes which we have observed. There have been others, such as those at the Memorial Hospital in New York, who have studied groups of cancer patients over these years and the infection among them. Also as you know, in recent years there has been a great interest in the changes in infections that occur in patients who have organ transplants. In each instance we have a different set of circumstances, with a new class of microbes involved. I suppose we call them "infections of medical progress" or "diseases of medical progress".

ERICSSON: I would like to ask one simple question of Dr. KASS. May I take it from what you said that you believe that people with gram-negative bacteremia may not run a fever ?

KASS: Absolutely.

ERICSSON: Well, I presume that you have proved that this is the case. I would like also to say that our general impression is much more like the one in Edinburgh than the one in Boston. We have a 2,000 bed hospital and in Sweden there is hardly anything which could be compared with a private hospital in the United States, so we think we have the whole population. But there is also one exception, which is probably quite evident to those of our American colleagues who had the opportunity to meet with us in Sweden lately and that is, patients infected outside the hospital do not get into our hospital, they go into special clinics which are, in our case, not even situated in the same place. So in our experience with infection we take between 100 and 150 thousands cultures a year.

Our experience is mainly related to patients who originally came into the hospitals for other reasons than infections. However, I would like to say that I have always stated that the pattern of resistance or sensitivity in a hospital, or indeed in any environment, is the negative imprint of the use of antibiotics in that environment. I have not seen nor heard of any so concentrated and so good a presentation of reasons for that and how this has to be done as in the presentation which Dr. FINLAND has just given us. However, we have not been studying this all over the hospital. As I hope to be able to tell you tomorrow—we have just used one of the units where, as Dr. FINLAND said in his introductory remarks, these factors have been involved and that is the burns unit. We, however, do believe that this can happen and it is not something which should happen without any resistance on the part of the doctor. This is no now idea of mine. It has been our working hypothesis for many years and one I first presented internationally at the NIH as a sort of farewell lecture after I had been working there for a period of time. Dr. WERNER and I said that this was always true but we cannot do anything about it, and not just as MARK TWAIN said—"everybody is talking about the weather but nobody is do anything about it"! In this case we are talking about it and we should be doing something about it.

FINLAND: I was going to say, with respect to the first question, that many of our bacteremic patients who are afebrile are also stuporous and unresponsive; we wonder why they are not answering our questions. When we take a blood culture we find they have gram-negative bacteremia. That answers our questions in part. This is particularly true in very old people; some of them already have meningitis or are in shock.

KASS: One small additional point that Dr. ERICSSON and I discussed last night, in Sweden earlier this year and also in the States. One of the important studies that needs to be done in the future is the comparative assessment of different hospital practices and different hospital populations by the same team in order to remove technical questions, which right now we cannot do. We need international studies in which the same groups use the same criteria so that we can then get an answer. There are a number of other variables that we should consider. Dr. ERICSSON mentioned that, in Sweden and in many countries, certain patients are isolated apart from the general hospital. There are other factors, for example, in Sweden the rate of surgery and the number of surgeons proportionally is approximately one third of that of the United States. Such things may be quite relevant. There are many possibilities of this sort and only well designed studies can help us understand them.

GOULD: By another quick calculation—I think it is of interest that the number —the proportion—of positive cultures in Boston, from Dr. KASS's and Dr. FINLAND's remarks, seems to be one in ten which almost exactly fits the figure for Edinburgh—namely 95%; so that perhaps this eliminates one of the variables.

KASS: We have about 25,000 blood cultures which means that about 4 to 5% are positive.

PULVERER: May I make two remarks concerning streptococci! Have I understood you correctly that at the end of your review or survey there was a rise in the number of hemolytic streptococcal bacteremias? If so, could this be in relation to tetracycline resistance? Secondly you mentioned here that tetracycline resistance is associated with group B streptococci. We published it 3 years ago and again last year that we also found very remarkable correlation between group B and tetracycline resistance and that there has also been chloramphenicol resistance in hemolytic streptococci of group B.

FINLAND: I think we should just answer this and then go on to the next paper because we shall have opportunities to go through this again. To answer the questions specifically—I think most of the bacteremic group A hemolytic streptococcal infections that occurred in the last few years were hospital-acquired infections or occurred in patients who came into the hospital from nursing homes with other serious conditions. In other words, these are a different kind of group A hemolytic streptococcal infections from the type that we saw in the early part of this study, which were mostly in people with primary streptococcal sepsis.

Group B is another special kind of infection involving mostly women or mostly babies and again it is a specific type. As to tetracycline resistance, incidentally, Dr. SABATH in the Channing Laboratory has recently confirmed the occurrence of tetracycline resistance in pneumococcus for the first time in our hospital. It has been shown, of course, in other places, that tetracycline resistant pneumococci do occur and may be quite common, as are group A hemolytic streptococci resistant to tetracyclines. We recently showed that some group B streptococci may also be resistant to tetracyclines.

SHOOTER: May I ask Dr. KASS whether he is going to do anything about this rise or does he really regard it like the weather, about which nothing can be done?

KASS: We are always trying to do something about it!

Bayer-Symposium III, 25—29 (1971)
© by Springer-Verlag 1971

The Changing Pattern of Infecting Organisms

S. Wysocki and H.-U. Drüner

With 7 Figures

The effectiveness of antibacterial chemotherapy is impaired by two mechanisms:
1. The acquired bacterial resistance of antibiotic sensitive bacteria.
2. The changing pattern of organisms from sensitive to resistant bacteria.

Hemolytic streptococci and pneumococci, which do not develop resistance, have lost most of their clinical importance ever since antibacterial agents were introduced into therapy. As the result of the widespread use of antibiotics they were replaced by resistant staphylococci which led to the problem of nosocomial staphylococcus infections. Newer antibiotics, effective against resistant staphylococci reduced the incidence of infection by this organism and made its treatment easier. Its place, however, was rapidly taken by resistant gram-negative bacteria. Of all gram-negative germs, *Pseudomonas aeruginosa* and Aerobacter/Klebsiella have become the most serious problem in the antibacterial treatment of surgical infections.

Hospital-acquired infections with organisms, which until now were considered to be of little or no pathogenic significance, have gained increasing importance in the last few years. Above all, in premature infants and in patients undergoing immunosuppressive therapy, an increased rate of severe infections with bacteria such as *Staphylococcus albus* or *Serratia marcescens*, as well as fungi, especially *Candida albicans*, are now observed.

In order to control these trends, it is necessary to register all infecting organisms which have been isolated. A survey in the hospital of over 25,000 different bacteria isolated from the wards of the Department of Surgery of the University of Heidelberg, 1959 to 1970, also shows a change in the pattern of the infecting organisms.

When comparing the patterns of *all* isolated germs, one recognizes that from 1965 to 1970 there has been an increasing incidence of gram-negative and a marked decrease in gram-positive bacteria. Urine cultures are not included in this diagram. Whilst in 1955, 30% of all pathogenic bacteria were staphylococci, the figure for 1970 is 22.8%; the corresponding figures for non-hemolytic streptococci were 12 and 7%.

The percentage of *Escherichia coli* and of Proteus shows a slight increase, whereas there is a significant increase of Aerobacter/Klebsiella and *Pseudomonas aeruginosa*. These two types of bacteria represent a combined incidence of more than 30% of all isolated bacteria.

In urine cultures, staphylococci are less frequent, whereas *Pseudomonas aeruginosa* is of increasing importance. *E. coli* are increasing slightly, whilst non-hemolytic streptococci remain about the same, Aerobacter/Klebsiella showing a decreasing incidence.

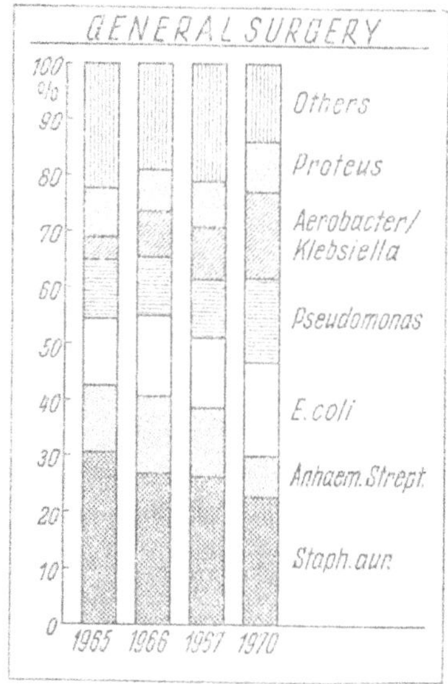

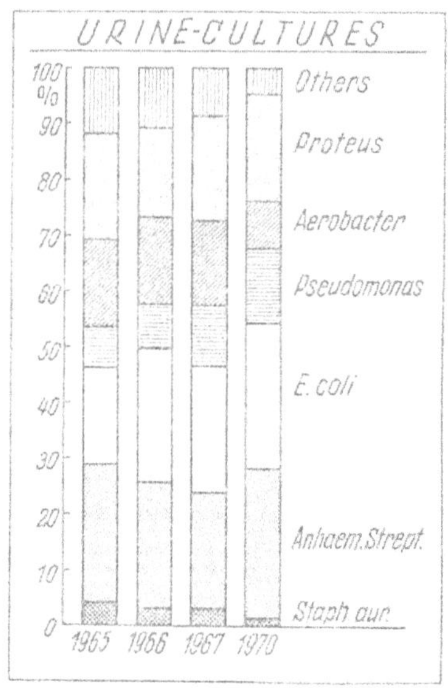

Fig. 1   Fig. 2

Fig. 1 The pattern of infecting organisms 1965—1970 (urine cultures are not included)

Fig. 2 The pattern of infecting organisms in urine cultures 1965—1970

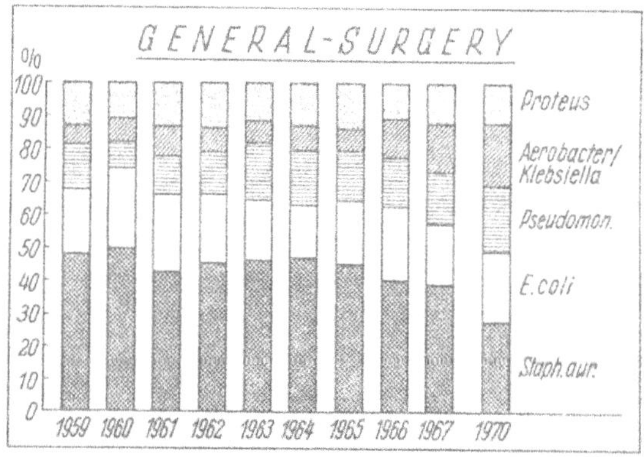

Fig. 3 The five most important infecting organisms 1959—1970 (urine cultures are not included)

Comparing the five most important infecting organisms—staphylococci, *E. coli*, *Pseudomonas aeruginosa*, Aerobacter/Klebsiella and Proteus—isolated from surgical patients, it becomes apparent that there is a continuous decrease in the proportion of staphylococci in the years from 1959 to 1970. Their share in 1959/60 was close to 50%, dropping to 29% in 1970. There is a striking increase of infections caused by *Pseudomonas aeruginosa* and Aerobacter/Klebsiella. In the group of the five most important bacteria they represent nearly 40%.

A survey of the same five bacteria isolated from urine cultures reveals an almost complete disappearance of *Staphylococcus aureus* and a growing threat by infections with *Pseudomonas aeruginosa*. Aerobacter/Klebsiella, which had shown a slight increase until 1967, was seen less frequently in 1970.

The majority of the urinary tract infections is caused by *E. coli* and Proteus. The change of the pattern of gram-positive to gram-negative bacteria took place at a steady rate. The development of resistance in the different types of bacteria varied periodically.

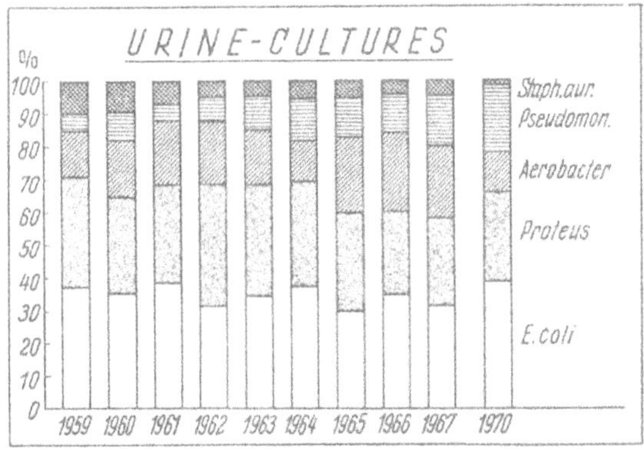

Fig. 4 The five most important infecting organisms in urine cultures 1959—1970

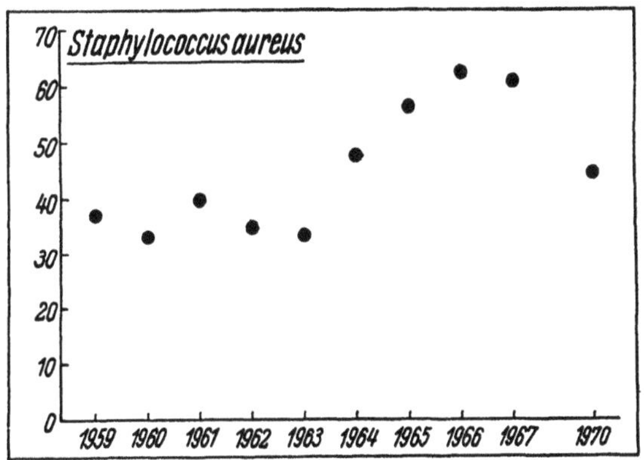

Fig. 5 Penicillin G — sensitivity of staphylocci isolated 1959—1970

Fig. 5 shows the sensitivity of all staphylococci isolated from patients of the Surgical Department of the University of Heidelberg since 1959. From 1959 to 1963 the proportion of sensitive strains was in the range of 30 to 35% and remained almost constant; from 1964 on there was an increase sensitivity, which continued until 1966 and 1967 when more than 60% of the staphylococci were sensitive to penicillin G. Early in 1970, however, our latest investigations showed a decrease in sensitivity to about 45%.

Since 1964, the indications for the application of antibiotics have been much more strict. At the same time the dosage for all antibiotics, especially for penicillin G, was raised, the maximum dose per day being given in every case of antibiotic therapy or prophylaxis, whereas in former years only minimum daily doses had been applied.

In Fig. 6 the relationship between the sensitivity of staphylococci to penicillin G and the average dosage of penicillin G in the individual patient is shown for the

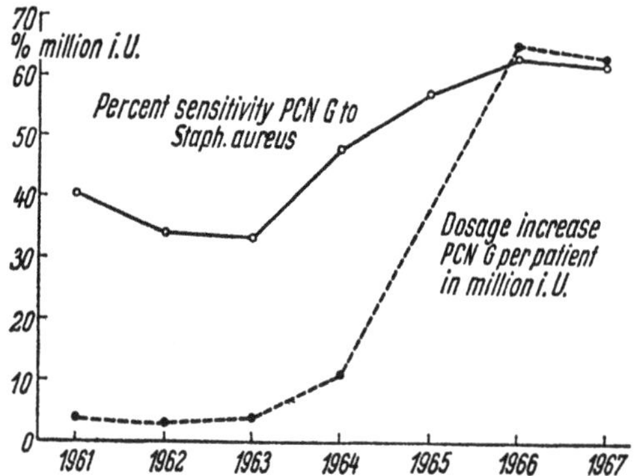

Fig. 6 Relationships between the penicillin G — sensitivity of staphylococci and the average dosage of penicillin G in the individual patient

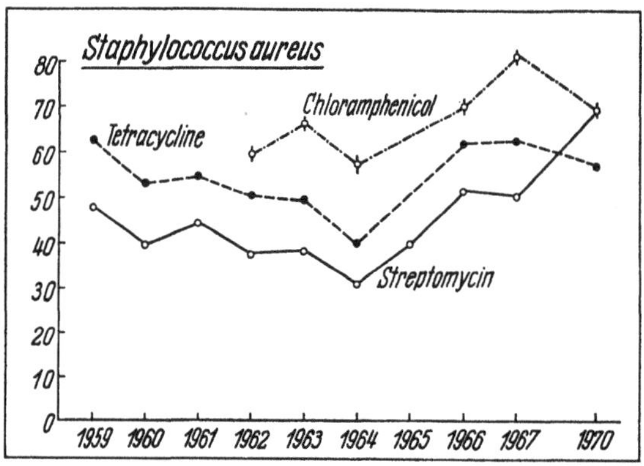

Fig. 7 Sensitivity of staphylococci to tetracycline, chloramphenicol and streptomycin 1959—1970

period of 1961 to 1967. The constant administration of higher doses of penicillin G seems to lower the incidence of resistant strains. In 1970, however, the proportion of staphylococci sensitive penicillin G was only 45%, although the dosage remained the to same.

As seen in Fig. 7, the same trend seems to hold true for tetracycline and chloramphenicol. Since 1964 streptomycin has no longer been administered at our hospital, except for tuberculosis. As a result there has been a continuous increase in the proportion of bacteria that are sensitive to streptomycin.

Serious problems in the application of effective antibacterial chemotherapy have been encountered in patients with a tracheostomy and longtime artificial respiration, as shown in Fig. 8. In the early sixties, after we started using long-term artificial respiration as a routine procedure, we were mainly concerned with respiratory infections caused by resistant staphylococci. In the following years, a new trend became apparent: the incidence of staphylococci became much lower in this group of patients: from 35% in 1966 to 12% in 1970.

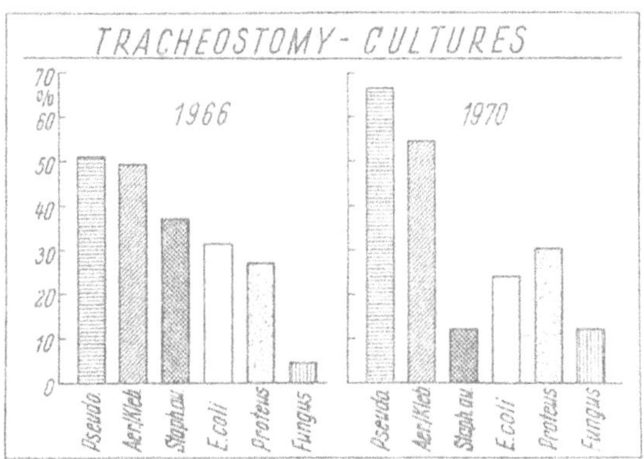

Fig. 8 Infecting organisms in patients with tracheostomy and long time artificial respiration

In 1966, as well as in 1970, we were alarmed by the large number of infections with Pseudomonas and Aerobacter/Klebsiella. In two-thirds of all cases, Pseudomonas, and in more than 50% Aerobacter/Klebsiella must now be taken into account. Very often mixed infections with both these organisms now represent a serious problem in antibacterial chemotherapy.

The incidence of *E. coli* and Proteus has not changed much. However, there has been a marked increase of infections with fungi. Septicaemia due to *Candida albicans* in adults was first observed at our hospital in 1970 in two patients who had prolonged treatment with high doses of various antibacterial agents. In both patients the septicaemia was preceded by an infection of the lung with *Candida albicans*. The change in the pattern of infecting organisms from sensitive to resistant types of organisms creates serious problems in patients with longterm artificial respiration. The question arises, therefore, whether in these cases intensive antibiotic therapy is useful at all, or whether such a therapy leads to an increasingly higher incidence of severe infections with resistant organisms and fungi.

Dr. S. WYSOCKI
Chirurgische Universitätsklinik
D-69 Heidelberg
Kirschnerstraße

Bayer-Symposium III, 31—35 (1971)
© by Springer-Verlag 1971

Etiology of Pyogenic and Urinary Tract Infections in the Region of Cologne

G. PULVERER, CH. GHO and CH. SPIECKERMANN

With 1 Figure

The spectrum of bacteria involved in infections is not constant. This relates not only to hospital infections but also to infections in general practice. During the last century we have seen at least three changes. The beginning of antisepsis/ asepsis caused one such change in spectrum. The introduction of sulphonamides and antibiotics in therapy brought about the next one. It now seems that another change in bacterial spectrum is occurring.

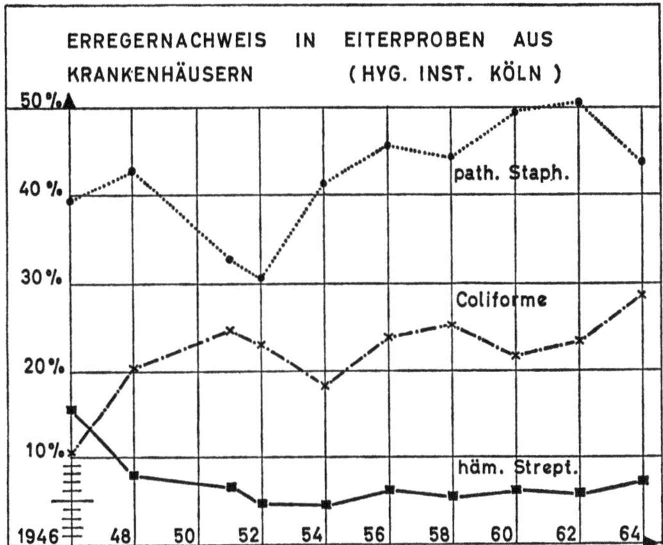

Fig. 1. Etiology of pyogenic infections in hospitals of the region of Cologne (PULVERER)

In 1959 FINLAND, JONES and BARNES reported on the material from the Boston City Hospital. They could demonstrate very impressively the changes from the time before sulphonamides to the era of antibiotics. Beta-hemolytic streptococci and pneumococci diminished, staphylococci and also the coliform group came into the foreground.

Five years ago we examined our material (PULVERER, see Fig. 1).

We included only hospital material which was sent to our institute for bacterial investigation, not only positive bacterial samples were encountered but also material which was shown to be sterile. Unfortunately, we have no data before 1946 because all documents in our institute were burned in 1945. Beta-hemolytic streptococci were relatively often identified in 1946, thereafter the percentage decreased. The frequency of coagulase-positive staphylococci in clinical material was already high in 1946. After 1948 there was a decline resulting, we believe, from the introduction of penicillin. After 1952 the percentage increased by about 20%. At that time the first broad spectrum antibiotics were introduced in Germany. From 1962 to 1964 there was again a fall, which may have been caused by the introduction of the new penicillins. By "coliforms" we mean aerobic gram-negative bacteria like *E. coli*, the Proteus-group, Aerobacter—Klebsiella and *Pseudomonas aeruginosa*.These coliform bacteria increased continuously from 1946 to 1964.

We reviewed our material once more. This time we iucluded only those specimens which yielded positive bacterial results. As we observed that the material from hospitals and from practice shows nearly the same spectrum, we considered all pyogenic infections examined at our institute. The percentages are, therefore, not comparable with those of our first study.

Table 1. *Gram-positive cocci in pyogenic infections*

Year	Samples examined	*Staph. aureus* %	*β*-hem. strept. %	*Strept. faecalis* %
1952	551	54	9	11
1954	604	70	10	12
1956	953	69	10	11
1958	1033	69	7	9
1960	1171	74	10	7
1962	1287	72	10	10
1964	1591	64	10	15
1966	1865	58	11	15
1968	1934	51	13	19
1969	4211	57	13	15
1970	1671	48	10	15

In Table 1 we compare the participation of the most important gram-positive cocci in cultures of pyogenic infections. As already seen in our first study, the rate for staphylococci decreased considerably after 1962. Beta-hemolytic streptococci remained constant at about 10%. To-date the increasing frequency of tetracycline-resistant streptococci did not influence these figures. The rate of enterococci, on the other hand, increased from 10 to 15%.

Table 2 shows the percentages of the most important gram-negative aerobic bacteria. *E. coli* and the Proteus-group exhibit moderately increasing proportions.

Very impressive is the rise of the Aerobacter/Klebsiella-group. In 1952 only 1 % of these bacteria was obtained from pyogenic infections; in 1970 the proportion was tenfold higher. Also *Pseudomonas aeruginosa* became a common agent in pyogenic lesions. The high rates of 1952 and 1958 were caused by hospital epidemics.

Table 3 demonstrates another very serious fact. Since 1952 not only the spectrum changed, that is, the gram-negative bacteria became more and more important, but the number of mixed infections increased markedly. During the years 1952 to 1954, 21% of the examined samples from pyogenic lesions were mixed infected; in 1969 it was 33% and in 1970 it was 26%. This clearly demonstrates the growing importance of the gram-negative bacteria.

Table 2. *Gram-negative bacteria in pyogenic infections*

Year	Samples examined	E. coli %	Aerobacter-Klebsiella %	Proteus sp. %	Pseudomonas aeruginosa %
1952	551	13	1	11	19
1954	604	12	2	8	3
1956	953	13	2	11	6
1958	1033	12	3	8	12
1960	1171	11	5	8	8
1962	1287	14	8	9	9
1964	1591	19	12	11	14
1966	1865	15	8	13	23
1968	1934	21	13	16	17
1969	4211	17	9	15	19
1970	1671	23	12	17	19

Table 3. *Mixed infections in pyogenic infections*

Year	Samples examined	Rate of mixed infections %
1952	551	21
1954	604	21
1956	953	21
1958	1033	23
1960	1171	21
1962	1287	26
1964	1591	32
1966	1865	33
1968	1934	35
1969	4211	33
1970	1671	26

In Tables 4, 5 and 6 we present the findings in urinary tract infections. Only urine samples positive for bacteria were counted and material from both hospital and practice are included. *S. aureus* and beta-hemolytic streptococci are not at all important agents of urinary tract infections. The rate for staphylococci remained constant, whereas the rate for beta-hemolytic streptococci doubled. Enterococci were found in 24% of samples during 1952, in 42% during 1959, and in 29%

during the first 6 months of 1970. Another interesting feature is the enormous increase in samples of urine diagnosed as infected. In 1969 we demonstrated that 30 times as many urine samples were infected as in 1952.

E. coli even now is the most frequent bacterium in urinary tract infections; the proportion has remained constant at about 60%. The frequencies of the Proteus-group and of *Pseudomonas aeruginosa* have increased. Very striking is the rise of the percentage of Aerobacter—Klebsiella. Today, Aerobacter/Klebsiella is cultivated four to six times more often from urinary tract infections than before 1956.

Taple 4. *Gram-positive cocci in urinary tract infections*

Year	Samples examined	*Staph. aureus* %	β-hem. strept. %	*Strept. faecalis* %
1952	498	8	1	24
1954	508	4	2	28
1956	911	4	1	23
1958	1471	8	1	22
1960	1528	10	1	19
1962	2256	12	2	28
1964	3821	8	3	26
1966	6398	10	3	29
1968	11838	6	4	37
1969	13426	6	4	42
1970	7347	6	4	29

Table 5. *Gram-negative bacteria in urinary tract infections*

Year	Samples examined	*E. coli* %	Aerobacter-Klebsiella %	Proteus sp. %	*Pseudomonas aeruginosa* %
1952	498	60	2	12	3
1954	508	47	3	15	5
1956	911	60	3	16	3
1958	1471	55	6	17	6
1960	1528	65	15	18	3
1962	2256	56	19	21	7
1964	3821	56	17	19	6
1966	6398	56	21	19	7
1968	11838	57	18	20	8
1969	13426	57	14	20	7
1970	7347	57	13	20	8

As Table 6 shows, the number of mixed urinary tract infections has also increased: the proportion of infections that were mixed in 1952 was 23%, in 1969 it was 42% and in 1970 it was 39%. This development reflects the present day problems of chemotherapy of urinary tract infections.

What factors are responsible for these changes in the spectrum of pyogenic lesions and of urinary tract infections? It is very difficult to find a satisfactory answer to this question. Without doubt, the use of antibiotics and the differing antibiotic-resistance of bacteria have some influence. Also an increase of virulence of bacteria must be considered. For example, during the era of antibiotics true epidemic strains of staphylococci occurred, which were not seen before. Host resistance must be discussed. The patient-material differs significantly from that of 30 or 40 years ago. Finally, the increase in the gram-negative bacteria could be related to the great environmental resistance of these bacteria, so these "opportunists" have really good chances to wait somewhere in the hospital for a proper host. But other problems concerned with the change of the spectrum cannot be interpreted satisfactorily at the moment.

Table 6. *Mixed infections in urinary tract infections*

Year	Samples examined	Rate of mixed infections %
1952	498	23
1954	508	25
1956	911	22
1958	1471	28
1960	1528	30
1962	2256	37
1964	3821	33
1966	6398	37
1968	11838	40
1969	13426	42
1970	7347	39

References

FINLAND, M., JONES, W. F., Jr., BARNES, M. W.: Occurrence of serious bacterial infections since introduction of antibacterial agents. J. Amer. med. Ass. **170**, 2188—2197 (1959).

PULVERER, G.: Aktuelle Probleme der Mikrobiologie bei entzündlichen Erkrankungen der Ohren und der oberen Luftwege. H. N. O. **14**, 133—138 (1966).

Prof. Dr. G. PULVERER
Direktor des Hygiene-Instituts
der Universität Köln
D-5000 Köln-Lindenthal
Fürst-Pückler-Str. 56

Bayer-Symposium III, 37—40 (1971)
© by Springer-Verlag 1971

The Change of Causative Agents in Wound Infection, Septicaemia and Meningitis in a 2000-Bed Hospital from 1957 to 1968

P. Naumann

With 4 Figures

Taking into consideration the results of bacteriological examinations during the last years, the impression was gained that the share of gram-negative bacteria among causative agents of wound infection, as well as of septicaemia, has increased, while at the same time staphylococcal infections are on the decline.

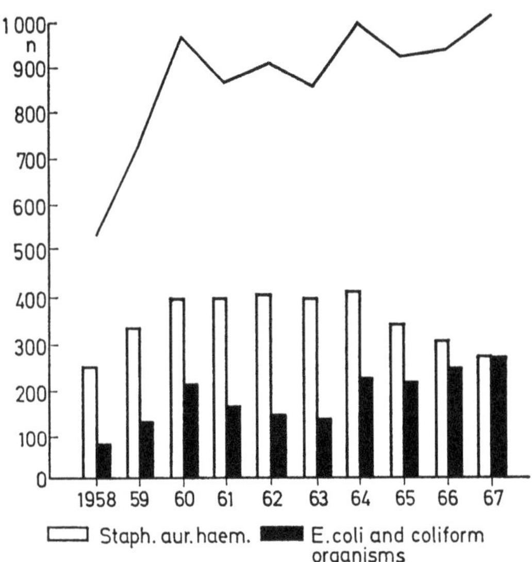

Fig. 1. Incidence of haemolytic staphylococci and *E. coli* together with other coliforms as causative organisms in wound infections from 1958 to 1967. The curve above the columns indicates the total number of all organisms isolated from wound infections

After the report of Fleming in 1968 on the same observations in Montreal, A. von Minckwitz and B. von Minckwitz have undertaken to sort and summarize the results of bacteriological examinations of material from the University Hospital of Hamburg-Eppendorf (a 2,000-bed hospital), and at the University Institute for Medical Microbiology and Immunology, Hamburg with regard to changes of causative agents from 1957 to 1968. Since 1963 we have observed a continuous decrease of coagulase-positive staphylococci as causative agents of wound infections from 46.6% (1963) to 26.6% (1967). On the other hand, during the same period the incidence of *Escherichia coli* and *coliform bacteria* as causative agents increased from 15.8% to 26.4%.

This change is shown in absolute numbers in Fig. 1; it demonstrates that *E. coli*, as well as other coliform bacteria, were isolated from wound infections just as frequently as haemolytic staphylococci. The increased percentage of the occur-

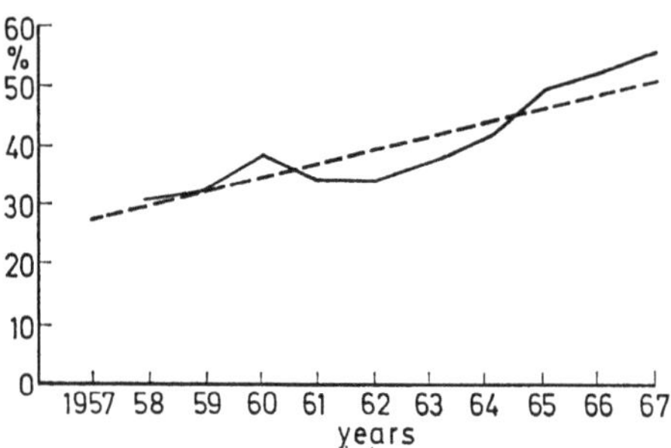

Fig. 2. Comparison of increase of gram-negative rods in wound infections from 1957 to 1967 in Hamburg (————) and in Montreal (- - - - -), the latter according to the data published by Fleming (1968)

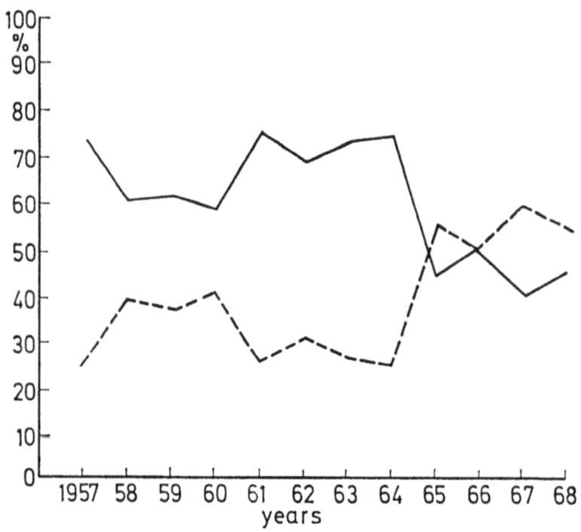

Fig. 3. Proportion (%) of gram-positive and gram-negative organisms as the causative agents in septicaemia (positive blood cultures) from 1957 to 1968 at the University Hospital, Hamburg-Eppendorf. ———— Gram-positive organisms; - - - - - gram-negative organisms

rence of *E. coli* and coliform bacteria in wound infections in the material from Hamburg corresponds exactly with the changes observed by Fleming in Montreal during the same period (Fig. 2).

This change occurred not only in wound infections but also in the distribution of the causative agents of septicaemia. Until 1964, the percent incidence of gram-positive organisms (haemolytic staphylococci, haemolytic streptococci, pneumococci and enterococci) in positive blood cultures had been 60 to 75%, it decreased by 1965 to 50 to 40%, while at the same time the frequency of gram-negative rods (*E. coli*, coliform bacteria, *Proteus* species and *Pseudomonas aeruginosa*) increased from 25% in 1964 to 50% in 1965 and 60% in 1968. Here also an increase in the absolute number of infections caused by the coli-group can clearly be recognized.

Figure 3 demonstrates the percent of gram-negative germs in septicaemia from 1957 to 1968 and it shows that since 1965 more gram-negative bacteria were isolated from blood cultures, than gram-positive ones.

Most surprising were the results of cerebrospinal fluid cultures. In 1960, gram-positive bacteria prevailed in more than 70% of the cases as the cause of bacterial meningitis (pneumococci, haemolytic streptococci and staphylococci) over gram-negative agents (meningococci, *Haemophilus influenzae* and *E. coli*) which con-

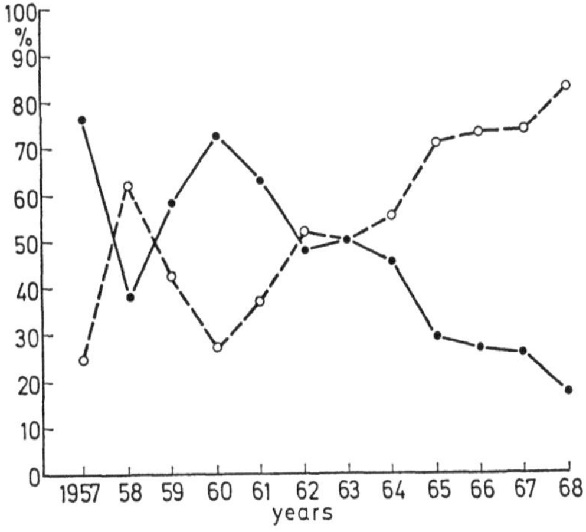

Fig. 4. Percent of gram-positive and gram-negative organisms in bacterial meningitis, isolated from 261 positive cerebrospinal fluid cultures from 1957 to 1968 (University Hospital, Hamburg-Eppendorf). ●—● Gram-positive organisms; ○—○ gram-negative organisms

stituted only 27% of the positive results. Since 1962, owing to the increased frequency of *E. coli* and other coliform bacteria, as well as the more frequent isolation of *Pseudomonas aeruginosa* and the unchanged frequency of meningococci and *Haemophilus influenzae*, a clear preponderance of gram-negative agents causing meningitis became manifest. In 1968, gram-negative bacteria accounted for 83% of all positive cerebrospinal fluid cultures, while gram-positive occurred in 17% only (Fig. 4).

Because the examined material had not been analysed according to the age groups of the patients, we cannot exclude the possibility that the cause of this change could be result of the more frequent examination of cerebrospinal fluid from newborn infants and children with a higher frequency of coli meningitis.

The material presented does not permit any conclusions as to the cause of the different distribution of gram-positive and gram-negative germs in wound infection, septicaemia and meningitis. It demonstrates, however, the whole-world trend during the last 6 to 7 years, namely, a distinct increase of frequency of gram-negative bacterial flora with simultaneous decrease of gram-positive organisms. This change is of great chemotherapeutic importance for the immediate treatment of a given case and should stimulate the search for antibiotics with special regard to their effectiveness against gram-negative bacteria.

References

FLEMING, D.: An epidemiological approach to control hospital infections with gram-negative bacteria. Int. J. Clin. Pharm., Therapy and Tox. 1, 397 (1968).

VON MINCKWITZ, A.: Erregerwandel bei Wundinfektionen von 1958 bis 1967 im Hamburger Raum (in preparation).

VON MINCKWITZ, B.: Häufigkeitsverteilung von Sepsis- und Meningitiserregern in Hamburg in den Jahren 1957 bis 1968 (in preparation).

Prof. Dr. P. NAUMANN
Institut f. med. Mikrob. u. Virologie
Universität Düsseldorf
D-4000 Düsseldorf 1
Moorenstraße 5

Discussion

FINLAND: In response to Dr. GOULD's question and Dr. ERICSSON's remarks it is interesting to see that qualitatively we have the same observations in many places and in different kinds of hospitals. As a matter of fact, in 1959, when we first published our material, it was thought that ours was a dirty hospital with "dirty" patients, "dirty" doctors and everything favouring a great deal of hospital infection. However, DAVID ROGERS published the results on a much smaller amount of material from a "clean" and very fancy hospital—a big marble palace on the East river in New York and the trend was exactly the same in that marble palace where it cost about six or eight times as much to hospitalize a patient than it did in the Boston City Hospital, where they had nurses all over the place, very fancy doctors who charged high fees, whereas our doctors got almost nothing for their services and where we got entirely different kinds of patients. So that, qualitatively, the problem is the same but quantitatively it has been very different.

Addressing Dr. WYSOCKI, I would like to make a remark about the increase in susceptibility of bacteria. This is especially true recently for staphylococci and it has been noted in many hospitals in the United States. I have indicated that this is also true in our hospital. There has been an increase in susceptibility in the hospital strains, particularly for those antibiotics which we have come to use less frequently, but there was an *increase* in resistance to those antibiotics which we were using more frequently, like kanamycin. For example, between 1965 and 1969 in our hospital we had a marked increase in kanamycin-resistant strains, whereas penicillin-resistance has been somewhat less frequent, perhaps related to the use of semi-synthetic penicillins and cephalosporins. At the same time we demonstrated an increase in resistance to penicillin, tetracycline and erythromycin in the community, where those antibiotics are being used more frequently.

With regard to Dr. Wysocki's mention of the occurrence *Candida*, I would like to say that there will appear in the December issue of Archives Internal Medicine, a report by Dr. Publio Toala, Dr. Schroeder and myself on the significance of the *Candida* that we are obtaining from our clinical material. This is a very important point because for the treatment of serious candida infection we have only very toxic antibiotics, primarily amphotericin B. It is, therefore, very important to know when *Candida* is producing a serious infection—even when we got it out of the blood—if we are to institute a treatment which is itself as serious as the treatment with amphotericin. We found, as have some of our colleagues in another hospital in Boston, that just invasiveness (i.e. candidemia) does not necessarily mean serious disease and that this invasiveness of the organism occurs primarily when you suppress most of the other bacteria and also have other factors that decrease resistance. As soon as you stop treating the patient intensively with multiple or broad spectrum antibiotics, *Candida* usually disappears from the cultures. In fact, if one examines those patients who have candidemia and die, only a small minority of them have invasive tissue disease that could be demonstrated to be due to *Candida* by careful study of the organs at autopsy. Therefore, we have to be very careful in how we manage the patients with candidiasis when that develops during antibiotic therapy of other infections.

One of the important features of the serious infections with *Candida* is the accompanying candiduria at the time when you have the candidemia. To be sure, when this is demonstrated (by direct smear of voided urine) it may be too late but, on the other hand, that is the only type of infection which has been found to be associated with significant tissue invasiveness of these organisms.

Perhaps Dr. Kass might be too modest, but I think we should probably give him much of the credit for the marked increase in the number of urinary cultures that have been reported, not only as mentioned by Dr. Pulverer, but all over the world. This has been increasingly recognised as an important factor in assessing the significance and the seriousness of bacterial infection of the urinary tract.

The increase in the cases of meningitis with gram-negative bacilli is interesting, and I would like to ask Dr. Naumann whether he has a breakdown of his cases by age, because in our hospital gram-negative meningitis, although not limited to the newborn period, is primarily a disease of newborn infants? It has been occurring somewhat more frequently in adults but, as with bacteremia, so with meningitis, the number of cases of meningitis due to pneumococcus has not changed over the years, and staphylococcal meningitis is still an extremely rare disease, even in our hospital. Meningitis due to gram-negative bacilli, except in newborns and as a terminal event in some of our patients with gram-negative bacteremia, is still very uncommon.

Williams: I fancy that I detect a fallacy in the way in which many of the statistics relating to number of infections are being presented. So far we have been shown changes in the proportion of cultures that yield particular bacteria. Now Dr. Pulverer mentioned that a large proportion of the infections are mixed infections. If we are going to talk about the frequency of infections with particular organisms or changes in the frequency over the years, we must refer to *patients*.

Individual patients may have 1, 2 or 3 cultures made from their wounds and each culture may grow 1, 2 or more different organisms. I think that we are very liable to be misled if we equate changes in the proportion of particular *organisms* in cultures to changes in the proportion of *patients infected* with different organisms. In our experience some 25 to 30% of patients with surgical wound infections have both a *Staphylococcus aureus* and a coliform organism in the wound at one time or another; if *Staphylococcus* is more easily eliminated by antibiotics than the coliform, those patients who have two successive cultures are likely to have a predominance of cultures yielding coliform bacteria. As the antibiotics effective against gram-positive bacteria have increased in effectiveness over the years, we should necessarily have seen an increase in the proportion of cultures yielding coliforms organisms, but that proportion of patients with infections caused by coliform organisms may not really have changed at all. It may be true that the greatest problem in the treatment of surgical infections now is the gram-negative organism, but the change in this direction over the years is due to increasing ease of treating the gram-positives; it is not necessarily true to say that there has been a change in the proportion of infections primarily caused by these organisms.

REBER: We can confirm Dr. FINLAND's observations that *Candida* disappears frequently from washed sputum flecks soon after stopping chemotherapy, in which case the bacterial equilibrium is disturbed by antibiotics. Giving oral chemotherapy causes disappearance of the *Candida* from the intestine. But a second possibility for diminishing diagnosis of *Candida* is technical. One condition is to *isolate Candida* rapidly from the sputum. For example, 4 h after obtaining the sputum and before it is cultured, we have an accumulation of *Candida* in the sputum which can result in the false diagnosis of candidiasis. After 6 h at room temperature we have seen multiplication from 1 to 50 times. *Candida* also often disappears only after antifungal treatment. In such cases it seems that the point from which dissemination occurs is the intestinal tract; if the organisms at this source are eliminated they no longer become fixed to other tissues. Turning to Dr. WYSOCKI's point, infection of tracheostomies is now commonly observed in hospitals. The most frequent sources are the humidifiers, and safe types are difficult to obtain. The lack of bacterial filters in inhalation apparatus or contamination by direct contact from nurses' hands while caring for the tracheostomies may also be important. What does Dr. WYSOCKI consider to be the main reason for this high infection rate ?

VON GRAEVENITZ: Without disputing what has been said before, I should like to discuss the question of mixed infections. We have found that if one uses media that are inhibitory for gram-negative rods, like Elmer's colymycin-nalidixic acid agar and Staphylococcus medium 110 or Chapman-Stone agar, the percentage of gram-positives does actually become higher in mixed infections than if you just use blood-agar and an agar for gram-negative rods like McCONKEY or dexoxycholate agar. The difference was as high as 15% in a comparative series, although I do not have the exact figures.

WYSOCKI: Dr. REBER asked about the manner of infection in tracheostomies. We tried to avoid this infection with all kinds of aspetic treatment but we could not do much and we could not prevent these infections. You may gain some time, but after prolonged artificial respiration, you have these infections any way.

NAUMANN: Dr. FINLAND, you asked me about the age of patients and the number of cases of gram-negative bacillus meningitis. I cannot answer this question because the results of our investigations of changes of the infecting organisms are not related to certain age groups. However, it is possible that this increase is caused by a large number of specimens of cerebrospinal fluid after neurosurgical measures. We obtained much more material in the second half of our observation period from the neurosurgical hospital. Perhaps that is the reason.

PULVERER: In reply to Prof. WILLIAMS' question, in my lecture I gave only data related to samples and not to patients. It was impossible to get the exact patient-data for every year. Nevertheless, I think that our material reflects the real situation because of several reasons: since 1952 the methods used in our laboratory are identical; the ratio of patient cultures in 1952 and in 1970 was very similar as we checked at random. Also the chance for secondary contamination during all the years was surely the same. Therefore it is my impression that there was really a rise in mixed infections. I cannot give an exact interpretation for this. Of course the gram-negative bacteria are not so virulent as, for example, the staphylococci. Therefore, I believe that these opportunists need the help of other bacteria to start or to sustain an infectious process.

FINLAND: The problem raised by Dr. WILLIAMS is a very important one, it is one that has bothered me since I began getting together our own data. Back in 1934[1], I gave my first report on "mixed infections" in pneumococcal pneumonia and at that time there were three kinds of mixed infections. When we tried to determine, by the best methods available, the relationship of the organisms that we cultivated from infections in the patients, we found that there were: (1) concomitant or concurrent infections where patients come in with both organisms producing disease; (2) consecutive infections, where one infection is present first and then another one supervenes and (3) infections in which one organism is actually producing disease and for the other we cannot document disease, that is, the other organisms are incidental. We made another study with Dr. TILLOTSON more recently with respect to pneumonias admitted to our hospital in which consecutive patients were studied serially from the time of admission. All of the data are not yet available because the studies of the serological response of the patients are not complete. This is one of the parameters that must be considered in trying to correlate isolation of bacteria with disease in the patient.

On the basis of sputum cultures, we tried to rate the organisms and the evidence of infection by: (1) the cytological response in the sputum; (2) whether the organism is found in pure culture or as the predominant one and (3) whether it is associated with an inflammatory response, as evidenced by fever and massive numbers of polymorphonuclears in the sputum. When these conditions were satisfied, we considered that as evidence of infection. Where the original causative organism declined or disappeared from the sputum and another one appeared,

---

[1] FINLAND, M.: The significance of mixed infections in pneumococcic pneumonia. J. Amer. med. Ass. **103**, 1681—1686 (1934).

even if it is increased in number, but there was no evidence of changes of the infection in the patient, that is, if there was no return of fever and symptoms and no return or change back to a large number of polymorphonuclears in the sputum, we could consider that as "colonization" rather than "infection". We tried to make that distinction which I think is important[2].

The same is also true in bacteriuria and in urinary tract infections; if you find small numbers of other bacteria that might not be significant and if they are not associated with other evidence of infection, we would not consider them as important. So we have to consider the patients, the organisms and the relation of those organisms to the evidence of infection in the patient.

Another point referred to is the use of differential media, the kind of primary media used and the number of types of media. This, too, may be an index of how many organisms you can culture and how one can miss recognizing even highly pathogenic organisms within the patient. This was very clearly brought home to us the time when we first recognized the syndrome of enterocolitis due to *Staphylococcus*. In our hospital, as I suppose in most hospital bacteriology laboratories, the tradition has been to culture faeces on a medium that would bring out pathogenic gram-negative bacilli. These media are also exactly the ones that will suppress gram-positive bacteria, particular staphylococci. However, when we merely made a smear of the watery stool, and looked at it with a gram stain, some of these specimens from patients with the marked watery diarrhoea showed only or predominantly staphylococci and no gram-negatives; there were also numerous leukocytes so that we were sure we were dealing with a true infection. All we had to do then was to make cultures on blood-agar plates and they showed almost pure cultures of staphylococci.

This is also an important aspect of the changes in the organisms occurring in tracheostomy cases. This has been studied in many areas and was part of Dr. TILLOTSON's study too. Incidentally in that study the importance of excessively large doses of penicillin was also brought out. It was shown that when we used more than 3 million IU/day of penicillin or 3 g of ampicillin to treat pneumococcal infections, there was a statistically greater chance of getting colonization and infection with gram-negatives than when smaller doses were used. The other point was the question of avoiding this change or treating it, and whether to use systemic or inhalation therapy. That classical study of Dr. LOUIS WEINSTEIN in patients who were subjected to tracheostomy following poliomyelitis, and also a similar study done by Dr. LEPPER and his associates in Chicago, showed that, regardless of whether you used 1, 2, 3, 4 or 5 antibiotics, the only thing you prevent and suppress is the organisms which are susceptible to those antibiotics. Invariably they ended up with the multiplication of organisms which were resistant to exactly the single or multiple antibiotics which were administered but they did not prevent infection by those other organisms, even when they gave multiple antibiotics, systemically or by aerosol.

---

[2] TILLOTSON, J. R., FINLAND, M.: Bacterial colonization and clinical superinfection of the respiratory tract complicating antibiotic therapy of pneumonia. J. infect. dis. **119**, 597—624 (1960).

DASCHNER: The very high incidence of mixed infections in urinary tract infections reported by Dr. PULVERER may have been due to contamination before the specimen reached the laboratory. Since we introduced the suprapubic bladder aspiration for routine diagnosis, the incidence of mixed infections dropped from between 20 and 30% down to between 1 and 5%.

KASS: The general problem, as Dr. FINLAND discussed it, is that of interpreting the results of the cultures. In interpreting cultures of urine, as Dr. DASCHNER has indicated, only two methods are available for telling contamination from true infection. One is quantitative bacteriology and the other is suprapubic aspiration. Quantitative bacteriology is much easier and lends itself to large scale work. As long as the specimen is transported promptly to the laboratory or is properly re-frigerated, the reliability compared to suprapubic puncture is almost 100%; the two correlate exceedingly closely. We do not advocate suprapubic aspiration except for special purposes because it is not necessary, but it is a reliable and more expensive way to do the job.

The point that emerges from the analysis of the data that have been collected with quantitative bacteriology is that the rate of mixed infection becomes low, the rate of infections to *Streptococcus faecalis* becomes very low and the rate of infection by staphylococci and by non-group A or other streptococci also fall to very low levels. One can use, as a rough rule, that when there are apparent in-fections with *Streptococcus faecalis*, other streptococci or other organisms of this group which are the common contaminants of the urethra, and these rates rise about 1%, it is almost certain evidence either that the cultures were not done quantitatively or that the cultures were stored under conditions in which the organisms could multiple in vitro. So I would have to suggest, as did Dr. DASCHNER, that the data on the urinary infections were probably collected with qualitative methods and without special care in cleansing. I would think, therefore, that the discussion on mixed infections and of enterococcal infections in the urinary tract should be held in abeyance.

In addition, we cannot evaluate the other areas of infection for the same reasons. In the urine we have a method for performing the evaluation of the cultures but in the other areas we do not yet have adequate methods.

In evaluating tracheostomies, we know there are normally no bacteria in the deeper bronchi: The bacterial content of the bronchial tree decreases rapidly below the carina. Therefore if a small plastic catheter is inserted below the carina and organisms are found, these are almost always present in high numbers, so that crude quantitation is useful in telling the difference between contamination by organisms that are not pathogenetically relevant and organisms that are in an area where organisms usually are not found and are, therefore, more likely to be involved in disease. We have only this one method for studying the pulmonary tree and it is limited in its usefulness. We have good methods for the urinary tract but for other areas of infection we really do not have reasonable methods for determining which organisms matter and which do not.

REBER: Up to now we have only discussed aerobic infections: what about anaerobes ? Dr. FINLAND, have you any interpretation of the fact that antibiotics are not only ineffective in prevention but can also frequently favour the infection as Johnston has demonstrated ? In clean operations he found three times as many infections with the use of antibiotic prophylaxis as compared with the rate in the series without antibiotics.

FINLAND: With respect to the last point, we have a constant battle with the surgeons and, in fact, with all physicians, on the problem of the use of so called prophylactic antibiotics, particularly to prevent diseases that are not there or those that you have no reason to believe should be there. There is no doubt in my mind that such use is bad, although the data for the proof are conflicting as to whether there is any true prevention or actual increase in infection with the use of prophylactic antibiotics. It is interesting in this regard that at a recent conference on hospital-acquired infections, a participating surgeon presented data indicating that when cephalordine was given just before and immediately after operations—clean operations—he had practically no post-operative infection, whereas if he did not use this drug he had, in the same hospital, a sizeable number of post-operative infections. However, when he was asked "Well, do you use this prophylaxis in your practice routinely" ? he said "No!, I do not use it. This was only a study .In my own operations I do not give any prophylactic antibiotics".

This is the point that I make and have made over the years and one which the late Prof. SAM HARVEY of Yale mentioned, also Dr. WANGENSTEEN of Minnesota stresses, that the use of antibiotics prophylactically has been a deterrent to the continued vigilance and care which good surgeons should exercise in their aseptic technique. Dr. WANGENSTEEN put it this way: "Prophylactic antibiotics might make a second rate surgeon out of a third rate surgeon, but it will never make a first rate surgeon out of a second rate surgeon". The late Prof. SAM HARVEY of Yale, in one of his lectures before he retired, indicated that the most important feature of the prevention of infections was the attention to strict asepsis during operations and that the use of antibiotics for prevention has not really improved the situation but has actually made it worse.

ERICSSON: May I first say in relation to the first papers, that there is a certain tendency to identify "parallelism or association of events" with "cause". There have been changes and there are certain changes in the pattern of infections which are not related to the use of antibiotics. For instance, I have been told by my earlier teachers that from the late 1930's or during the 1920's there was an obvious decrease in the rate of severe infections caused by beta-haemolytic streptococci, at least in Stockholm. It can also be indicated that there has been an increase of certain infections caused by highly sensitive micro-organisms. Of course, the excuse for the increase of the gonococcal infection is, at least in some peoples mind, the decrease in morals of young people and I do not think that this is an epidemiologic approach to the problem. However, let us speak about other bacteria, for example, meningococcus which, at least in our country, is increasing even though the organisms are all highly sensitive to many of the antibiotics which are used. May I also say to Dr. FINLAND that when you compared the incidence of infections in hospitals, hand washing is certainly not done with marble, but the soap and the hand washing are not parallel to the amount of marble in a hospital. I think that is so. We then credited Dr. KASS for having created the high frequency of the urinary tract infection but, as was evident from his last contribution to the discussion, I think, that Dr. KASS should be given just as much credit for pointing out that urinary tract infections are very often over-diagnosed and I thought that they were. It should be almost natural or self evident that any studies on frequency of urinary tract infections made after what Dr. KASS presented "the Kass-criteria for urinary tract infections" which do not use those criteria, can not be considered reliable, and statistics which do not adhere to those criteria should not be presented. Therefore, I do not believe in *Staphylococcus* as a cause of infections in the urinary tract, with very few exceptions and only under "septic" conditions. But I am also a little astonished, Dr. KASS, that you do not take the same approach to the problem of blood cultures. I think there is a certain tendency to over-diagnose the results of blood cultures and I come back to the discussion earlier this morning. We always make pour-plates with original blood and never regard as positive a single blood culture with gram-negative or any bacteria which are not found in the solid culture which is, of course, to a certain extent, a semi-quantitative procedure.

PULVERER: I know very well the dilemma when there are several different bacteria in one culture—which of these bacteria are responsible for the infectious process, which are only contaminants—especially with gram-negative bacteria. A reliable answer cannot be given in most cases. When I discussed the problem of "mixed" infections with surgeons, they told me that they prefer chemotherapy which shoots at all the bacteria.

As to Dr. DASCHNER's point, in Cologne we have very good contact with a surgeon in a large hospital. The doctors of this hospital send only catheter-urine, all samples are freshly collected and kept cool until cultured. So in these cases there is no chance for secondary contamination or multiplication. In this material we also found mixed infections in nearly the same percentages as given in the tables.

Bayer-Symposium III, 49—56 (1971)
© by Springer-Verlag 1971

Distribution of Pneumococcus Types at Different Times in Different Areas

Erna Lund

The pneumococci belong to the streptococcal tribe; they are gram-positive, capsulated diplococci, soluble in bile, and sensitive to optochin. They show alpha-haemolysis on blood agar and are virulent for mice.

Pneumococci are found especially in infections of the respiratory system, but are also present in bacteraemia, meningitis, peritonitis, and other infections. Capsulated and non-capsulated pneumococci can be isolated from the throat in about 50 % of healthy persons.

The pneumococci were first found by Pasteur in 1881. In 1909, the serologically different types 1 and 2 were described, followed soon after by type 3 and a group 4. About 1930, group 4 was divided into types 4 to 32. Later especially American and Danish workers have brought the number of pneumococcal types up to 82. During the last 4 years, we at Statens Serum-institut have been able to type all capsulated pneumococci. Thus. if more than 82 types exist, the rest must be rare or serologically very closely related to the known types.

In 1938, Statens Seruminstitut started production of therapeutic and diagnostic pneumo-coccal sera. In 1940, Kauffmann and co-workers reported 20 new pneumococcal types and carried out studies on the antigenic structure of the types. For practical reasons, related types were grouped together; for instance the 7-group consists of four serologically different types: 7F, 7A, 7B, and 7C, which have one or more antigens in common (Table 1).

This *Danish nomenclature* was discussed at the congress in Mexico August 1970, and I am told that there was no objection to its being used internationally.

The *diagnostic pneumococcal sera* produced at Statens Seruminstitut are type or group specific, covering the numbers up to 48 Numbers 26 and 30 are not used, since the types first called by these numbers were later found to belong serologically to group 6 and group 15.

For rapid diagnosis, we use a pooled concentrated serum, an *"Omni-serum"*, giving capsular reaction with all 82 types. Moreover, we have nine *pooled sera*, called by the letters A to I, together reacting with all types. For *type or group* diagnosis we have 46 sera, numbered from 1 to 48, numbers 26 and 30, as mentioned, not being used. The group sera and pooled sera are produced by immunization of rabbits with all types belonging to the group or pool.

The sera used for differentiation within the groups, the so-called *"factor-sera"*, are pro-duced only for our own laboratory. Most of these have low titres and can only be kept for a short time (Table 2).

Many authors have reported on the distribution of *Pneumococcus* types in lobar pneumonia (Table 3). Here are a few examples: In U.S.A., in 1913 type 1 was found in 47% and type 2 in 18%. The following year in the same hospital, type 1 was seen in 30% and type 2 in 39%, the change for type 2 in 1 year thus being from 18 to 39%. Other authors found similar figures, showing that type 2 varied greatly at different times and in different countries, while type 1 was relatively constant.

In South Africa, Lister found in 1913 to 1917 that type 5 was the most frequent type in pneumonia, namely 31%, while type 1 was seen in 22% and type 2 in 16%. Ordman continued these investigations and in 1938 reported type 1 in 22% and type 2 in 15%. The strong representation of type 5 had disappeared. Among the native miners type 2 dominated at that time.

Table 1. *Danish type designations of 82 pneumococci. Antigenic formulae according to* KAUFFMANN *and* LUND. *(Changed by* LUND. *1970)*

Type	Antigenic formula	Type	Antigenic formula
1	1a	20	20a, 20b, 7g
2	2a	21	21a
3	3a	22F	22a, 22b
4	4a	22A	22a, 22c
5	5a	23F	23a, 23b, 18b
6A	6a, 6b	23A	23a, 23c, 15c
6B	6a, 6c	23B	23a, 23b, 23d
7F	7a, 7b	24F	24a, 24b, 24d, 7h
7A	7a, 7b, 7c	24A	24a, 24c, 24d
7B	7a, 7d, 7e, 7h	24B	24a, 24b, 24e, 7h
7C	7a, 7d, 7f, 7g, 7h	25	25a, 25b
8	8a	27	27a, 27b
9A	9a, 9c, 9d	28F	28a, 28b, 16b, 23d
9L	9a, 9b, 9c, 9f	28A	28a, 28c, 23d
9N	9a, 9b, 9e	29	29a, 29b, 13b
9V	9a, 9c, 9d, 9g	31	31a, 20b
10F	10a, 10b	32F	32a, 27b
10A	10a, 10c, 10d	32A	31a, 32b, 27b
11F	11a, 11b, 11e, 11g	33F	33a, 33b, 33d
11A	11a, 11c, 11d, 11e	33A	33a, 33b, 33d, 20b
11B	11a, 11b, 11f, 11g	33B	33a, 33c, 33d, 33f
11C	11a, 11b, 11c, 11d, 11f	33C	33a, 33c, 33e
12F	12a, 12b, 12d	34	34a, 34b
12A	12a, 12c, 12d	35F	35a, 35b, 34b
13	13a, 13b	35A	35a, 35c, 20b
14	14a	35B	35a, 35c, 29b
15F	15a, 15b, 15c, 15f	35C	35a, 35c, 20b, 42a
15A	15a, 15c, 15d, 15g	36	36a, 9e
15B	15a, 15b, 15d, 15e, 15h	37	37a
15C	15a, 15d, 15e	38	38a, 25b
16	16a, 16b, 11d	39	39a, 10d
17F	17a, 17b	40	40a, 7g, 7h
17A	17a, 17c	41F	41a, 41b
18F	18a, 18b, 18c, 18f	41A	41a
18A	18a, 18b, 18d	42	42a, 20b, 35c
18B	18a, 18b, 18e, 18g	43	43a
18C	18a, 18b, 18c, 18e	44	44a, 44b, 12b, 12d
19F	19a, 19b, 19d	45	45a
19A	19a, 19c, 19d	46	46a, 12c, 44b
19B	19a, 19c, 19e, 7h	47	47a, 35a, 35b
19C	19a, 19c, 19f, 7h	48	48a

In Denmark in 1923, CHRISTENSEN found type 1 in 33% of cases of lobar pneumonia, and type 2 in 27%. Comparing these findings with the results of NISSEN in 1937, it was seen that type 2 had decreased from 27 to 1.7%, type 1 being the most frequent in both years with 33 and 40%.

In Norway in 1940, BJØRNSSON found type 1 in 22% and type 2 in 1%. The same year VAMMEN in Denmark saw type 1 in 21% and type 2 in 2%.

Table 2. *Pneumococcal factor sera*

Type	Antigenic formula	Factor sera				
		6b	6c			
6A	6a, 6b	+	−			
6B	6a, 6c	−	+			
		7b	7c	7e	7f	
7F	7a, 7b	+	−	−	−	
7A	7a, 7b, 7c	+	+	−	−	
7B	7a, 7d, 7e, 7h	−	−	+	−	
7C	7a, 7d, 7f, 7g, 7h	−	−	−	+	
		9b	9c	9d	9e	9g
9A	9a, 9c, 9d	−	+	+	−	−
9L	9a, 9b, 9c, 9f	+	(+)	−	−	−
9N	9a, 9b, 9e	+	−	−	+	−
9V	9a, 9c, 9d, 9g	−	(+)	+	−	+
		10b	10c			
10F	10a, 10b	+	−			
10A	10a, 10c	−	+			
		11b	11c	11f		
11F	11a, 11b, 11e, 11g	+	−	−		
11A	11a, 11c, 11d, 11e	−	+	−		
11B	11a, 11b, 11f, 11g	+	−	+		
11C	11a, 11b, 11c, 11d, 11f	−	(+)	+		
		12b	12c			
12F	12a, 12b, 12d	+	−			
12A	12a, 12c, 12d	−	+			
		15b	15c	15d	15e	15h
15F	15a, 15b, 15c, 15f	+	+	−	−	−
15A	15a, 15c, 15d, 15g	−	(+)	(+)	−	−
15B	15a, 15b, 15d, 15e, 15h	+	−	(+)	+	+
15C	15a, 15d, 15e	−	−	+	+	−
		17b	17c			
17F	17a, 17b	+	−			
17A	17a, 17c	−	+			
		18c	18d	18e	18f	
18F	18a, 18b, 18c, 18f	+	−	−	+	
18A	18a, 18b, 18d	−	+	−	−	
18B	18a, 18b, 18e, 18g	−	−	+	−	
18C	18a, 18b, 18c, 18e	+	−	(+)	−	

Table 2 (continued)

Type	antigenic formula	Factor sera			
		19b	19c	7h	19f
19F	19a, 19b, 19d	+	−	−	−
19A	19a, 19c, 19d	−	+	−	−
19B	19a, 19c, 19e, 7h	−	(+)	+	−
19C	19a, 19c, 19f, 7h	−	(+)	+	+

Type	antigenic formula	22b	22c
22F	22a, 22b	+	−
22A	22a, 22c	−	+

Type	antigenic formula	23b	23c	28
23F	23a, 23b, 18b	+	−	−
23A	23a, 23c, 15a	−	+	−
23B	23a, 23b, 23d	(+)	−	+

Type	antigenic formula	24c	24d	24e
24F	24a, 24b, 24d, 7h	−	+	−
24A	24a, 24c, 24d	+	+	−
24B	24a, 24b, 24e, 7h	−	−	+

Type	antigenic formula	28b	28c
28F	28a, 28b, 16b, 23d	+	−
28A	28a, 28c, 23d	−	+

Type	antigenic formula	32a	32b
32F	32a, 27b	+	−
32A	32a, 32b, 27b	+	+

Type	antigenic formula	33b	20b	33f	33e
33F	33a, 33b, 33d	+	−	−	−
33A	33a, 33b, 33d, 20b	+	+	−	−
33B	33a, 33c, 33d, 33f	−	−	+	−
33C	33a, 33c, 33e	−	−	−	+

Type	antigenic formula	35b	35c	29b	42a
35F	35a, 35b, 34b	+	−	−	−
35A	35a, 35c, 20b	−	+	−	−
35B	35a, 35c, 29b	−	(+)	+	−
35C	35a, 35c, 20b, 42a	−	+	−	+

Type	antigenic formula	41a	41b
41F	41a, 41b	+	+
41A	41a	+	−

+ = capsular reaction, (+) = weak reaction.

In 1949, I published a work on the frequency of *pneumococcus* types in Denmark during the 8 years 1939 to 1947. I have made similar investigations for the last 15 years: 1955 to 1970. Type 1 has decreased from 13.1 to 1% and type 2 from 6 to 1.5%.

Table 4 shows a comparison between the most common types of pneumococci isolated from patients in the two periods just mentioned. In the first period, type 1 was most frequent in blood, spinal fluid, pleural exudate, and pus from ears; in sputum it was the second most frequent. During these years, types 2 and 6 were among the dominant types.

Table 3. *Distribution of pneumococcus types 1 and 2 in pneumonia to different times and in different areas*

Area	Year	Percentage	
		Type 1	Type 2
U.S.A.	1913	47	18
U.S.A.	1014	30	39
South Africa	1913—1917	22	16
Denmark	1923	33	27
Denmark	1937	40	1.7
South Africa	1938	22	15
Norway	1940	22	1
Denmark	1940	21	2
Denmark	1939—1947	13.1	6
Denmark	1955—1970	1.0	1.5

Table 4. *Comparison of the most common pneumococcal types in 1939—1947 and in 1955—1970*

Material	1939—1947							1955—1970						
Blood	1	2	3	6	4	12	23	14	4	1	7	3	23	9
Spinal fluid	1	3	6	18	2	4	19	18	14	7	6	3	23	19
Pleural exudate	1	2	6	3	19	7	8	3	23	1	14	19	9	7
Expectorate	3	1	2	7	6	19	8	6	19	3	23	9	17	15
Swabs	6	19	1	14	3	18	23	19	6	3	23	14	9	11
Ear	1	3	19	6	14	5	18	19	14	6	23	3	18	1
Sinus maxillaris[a]	6	3	19	23	22			6	23	19	8	34	18	7

[a] The material is from 1941—1947.

In the second period *i.e.* during the last 15 years, type 1 is not the most frequent in any material. In spinal fluids, sputum, and swabs from throat and sinus maxillaris, type 1 is not among the seven most frequent types.

Comparing the two periods, it will be seen that type 2 has changed a great deal. In 1939 to 1947, this type was one of the most common in blood, pleural exudate, and sputum, while in recent years, this type was not to be found among the seven most frequent types.

Table 5 gives the type distribution of 2,684 strains from different materials for the last 15 years. The types found in less than 1% are omitted. The seven most frequent types for the whole material are: 19, 6, 14, 23, 3, 7, 18. Type 1 is number 10 and type 2 number 19. Type 14 was found most frequently in blood, type 18 in spinal fluid, type 3 in pleural exudate, type 6 in sputum and pus from nose and sinus maxillaris. In swabs from throat, larynx, and ears, type 19 was dominant. On the whole, type 19 was the most frequent type.

Table 5. *Distribution of pneumococcus types in different materials 1955—1970 (2,684 strains). The types found in less than 1 % are omitted*

Type	Blood	Spinal fluid	Pleural exudate	Expect- orate	Swab	Ear	Nose	Total number	%	frequen- cy
1	44	14	15	4	4	19	3	103	3.8	10
2	8	20	7	6	2	1	—	44	1.6	19
3	37	46	18	34	24	32	9	200	7.4	5
4	45	31	3	5	3	2	2	91	3.4	11
6	29	52	8	41	42	35	38	245	9.1	2
7	38	53	9	12	12	12	10	146	5.4	6
8	29	42	8	12	8	15	14	128	4.8	8
9	30	28	10	27	15	8	10	128	4.8	9
10	5	9	6	9	7	6	3	45	1.7	18
11	7	8	2	11	15	1	10	54	2.0	16
12	23	21	1	3	2	4	2	56	2.1	14
14	50	56	15	14	16	50	7	208	7.7	3
15	10	13	6	18	14	11	8	80	2.9	12
16	3	6	3	8	3	4	6	33	1.2	21
17	9	4	2	21	5	6	8	55	2.0	15
18	19	61	5	7	15	21	11	139	5.1	7
19	26	44	14	36	51	94	27	292	10.8	1
20	7	5	4	5	3	1	6	31	1.2	22
22	14	9	8	14	5	1	1	52	1.9	17
23	32	45	16	29	22	34	28	206	7.6	4
31	3	2	5	10	6	—	1	27	1.0	24
33	8	10	2	5	2	1	1	29	1.1	23
34	4	14	6	18	12	—	12	66	2.4	13
35	2	4	5	7	10	—	7	35	1.3	20

Table 6 shows a list of pneumococcal types found in materials not mentioned in Table 5. Pneumococci were isolated from eyes in 26 patients, and from peritoneum and urine in eight specimens each. Moreover, pneumococci have been found in arhtritis, pericarditis, skin infections, and so on, as can be seen from the table. Pneumococci have, for instance, been isolated from bile, faeces, and intestines.

The pneumococci found in animals and in man are identical, and infection may be carried from animal to man, and vice versa.

The pneumococci have constant *virulence for mice* as long as the capsule formation is unchanged. I have transferred *Pneumococcus* cultures in serum broth 300 times at 37 and 41 °C and found no reduction in virulence, as long as the capsule reaction was optimal. Thus, the virulence depends on the capsule and is constant for the same type. All S (smooth) pneumococci are virulent for mice, but to varying degrees. R pneumococci—that is non-capsulated strains—are avirulent.

In mice and *in vitro*, it is possible to change one pneumococcal type into another.It has not been noted whether a change in type might take place in the human throat. By means of repeated and thorough examination of the *Pneumococcus* types in swabs from the throat, it is possible to find both capsulated and non-capsulated strains and in some cases several types in the same swab. It is therefore impossible to prove that one of the types found has been produced by a change in a type found previously.

Table 6. *Pneumococcal types found in different material (1955—1970)*

Specimen from	Number of patients	Pneumococcal types
Eye	26	3, 6, 6A, 6A, 8, 9, 9, 11A, 12, 14, 14, 17, 17, 18C, 19, 19, 21, 22, 23, 23, 23, 23F, 25, 34, 34, 37
Peritoneum	8	1, 3, 4, 9N, 11A, 12A, 15A, 37
Urine	8	8, 18, 19, 19A, 20, 23, 34, 35B
Joint	6	8, 8, 9V, 14, 18C, 25
Bone-marrow	1	9
Pericardium	2	3, 15B
Skin infection	6	3, 6, 6, 6B, 14, 17F
Abscess	4	4, 6, 7, 9
Cicatrice	4	6B, 7, 8, 9N
Stomach	4	8, 14, 15, 33A, 35A
Gall bladder	2	9, 23F
Duodenum	1	18C
Intestine	1	1
Appendix	1	39
Faeces	1	6B
Uterus	1	31
Pus from ovary	1	23
Pus from drain	1	23
Abscessus ad anum	1	31
Total	79 specimens	

Finally, a few words about the diagnosis of pneumococci. Almost all strains are sensitive to *optochin*. Our *optochin test* is made with a 6 mm optochin disc of 10 µg placed on a blood agar culture. Pneumococci give a zone of inhibition of > 20 mm in diameter, while streptococci give no zone or < 15 mm. R pneumococci are sensitive to optochin.

The *bile test* on pneumococci is less reliable than the optochin test.

The *Neufeld test* shows the capsular reaction. A small amount of the specimen is placed on a slide and mixed with a loopful of serum only with antiserum against the same type. A coverslip is then placed on the mixture. Under the microscope, a positive reaction shows the capsule as a dark outline.

In an *India-ink* preparation, the capsule will be of the same size as in a positive Neufeld reaction.

After the introduction of *sulpha* preparations and especially of *penicillin*, treatment with type specific sera was discontinued and Statens Seruminstitut stopped producing pneumococcal sera, since no typing is necessary for antibiotic treatment.

Nevertheless, several laboratories requested us to resume the production of diagnostic sera. This we have done, and now still more institutions are using our sera.

References

LUND, E.: Laboratory diagnosis of pneumococcus infections. Bull. Wld Hlth Org. **23**, 5—13 (1960).

— Die Pneumokokkeninfektion: Die Infektionskrankheiten des Menschen und ihre Erreger, S. 667—679. Stuttgart Thieme 1969.

— On the nomenclature of the pneumococcal types. Int. J. syst. Bact. **20**, 321—323 (1970).

Futher references can be found in the papers quoted here.

Dr. ERNA LUND
Statens Seruminstitut
Amager Boulevard 80
DK-2300 Kopenhagen S

Discussion

FINLAND: This represents a tremendous and continuous effort. We are all grateful to Dr. LUND for continuing these efforts. Those of us who have been interested in the pneumococcus for many years are particularly indebted because the only source of reliable material is from her laboratory.

I would like to start the discussion by posing a question which was raised during a recent discussion in the vaccine therapy committee in the United States. We should have had you, Dr. LUND with us! They were considering the development of a polyvalent vaccine containing the antigenic type-specific polysaccharides of the 5, 6 or 7 most common pathogenic types. From your observations —epidemiological and serological—do you feel that such a vaccine has any merit?

LUND: I feel it is impossible to say what such a vaccination will do until you have tried it. As compared with the immunisation of rabbits, we have to immunise them three times per week for 3 to 4 weeks until we get serum of reasonable titre. I think that with only one injection in the human-being it is very doubtful if it will have enough effect. But the future will tell.

KASS: Were the two strains pneumococci from the gall bladder bile-soluble?

LUND: We almost never use the bile test.

FINLAND: I would like to answer that question because we have encountered some such strains and they are bile soluble. There was no effective bile in those gall bladders because they were diseased gall bladders and had a lot of pus, but no bile.

LUND: Ours was a pure culture isolated from another laboratory, so it was alive.

WILLIAMS: Does Dr. LUND have any idea as to why there has been the change in type distribution? Why do we now see fewer type 1's than we used to?

Lund: I think it is a part of the same problem which you have discussed with regard to age; we have more older people. There are certain types we culture especially from children and others from older people. I think that it is exactly the types that affected people between 20 and 40 years old who are now treated and cured and those types are less common. However, the older people do not have the same resistance and they develop infection with the same types as before.

Williams: May I come back to my question. Are you suggesting that there is really no change in the frequency with which type 1 infects people but merely that there is a change in the frequency with which laboratories receive pneumococci from the people infected with type 1 ?

Lund: I do not know.

Finland: May I interject that Dr. Robert Austrian of Philadelphia, in connection with his vaccine project, recently visited some of the places in South Africa where the original strains were first serotyped and classified. They still have type 1 and type 2 in approximately the proportions that they had before. The patients there are people that come by contract from the bush-country.They are the negroes who come to the compounds in the mines and live in very close contact with each other; they still have type 1 and type 2 pneumococci and some of the lower types which are infrequent with us in the United States. That does not explain why we do not have them but they are certainly less frequent in the United States than they are in Denmark.

In this connection it is interesting that there has been a very marked change in the occurrence and the pathogenicity of the specific groups of meningococci. As you know, during World War II there was an intensive study of meningococcal infections, not only in the military but also in the civilian populations and by far the most frequent serotype has been group A. This group is now extremely rare except in North Africa. Most of the recent infections, as well as the carriers, have been with group B. However the predominant group now is group C and in some areas even group C is being seen less frequently. A new group, group Y, has recently been found in some places as the carrier strain although they have not been shown to be pathogenic until very recently when there have been isolated cases, so that this phenomenon of the shifting frequency of types is as true there as we find with pneumococci, and with phage types of staphylococci, and so on.

Ericsson: Dr. Lund made some remarks about the diagnosis of a pneumococcus. I actually started my career as a bacteriologist working with the typing of pneumococci but I must admit that I, and I think most bacteriologists in Sweden, have given up the typing and are now relying very much upon the optochin test, as you describe it. I would like to ask a question about the amount of optochin in the disc ? You obviously have a sort of semi-quantitative estimation of the inhibition and you use a high amount of 10 μg but we have found that if you use amounts of between 2 and 3 μg, you get no inhibition at all with bacteria other than pneumococci. Is that not possibly a sort of error of interpretation if you have a zone size around other bacteria than pneumococci ?

LUND: The other bacteria can only be the non-hemolytic streptococci. There is a gap between the pneumococci and the streptococci. If you repeat it with a diluted culture you will not be in any doubt, and if you really are, I then recommend that you put the disc on the plate and take it off the next day, before you inoculate the plate; you will then get a zone about 30 to 35 mm with the pneumococci and no zone at all with the streptococci. That is 100% true.

PULVERER: During the last year we have found several tetracycline-resistant strains of pneumococci [Dtsch. med. Wschr. *92*, 1608 (1967)]. May I ask you if you have found some tetracycline-resistant strains that are resistant also to other antibiotics and if there is some correlation with serotypes?

LUND: In our department we only do the typing of pneumococci, we do not usually examine the sensitivity to antibiotics but we have received some strains, especially from Australia—from Dr. HANSMAN—and they were resistant to tetracycline. We have a few strains that are resistant to sulfonamide preparations, to streptomycin and other antibiotics but it is very seldom found. Some years ago I was in a department for antibiotics and from that time I have these strains. We have a museum of 200 different strains.

FINLAND: We have been doing susceptibility tests with available antibiotics on pneumococci on various occasions. We have never found any resistant strains to any antibiotics until this year when Dr. SABATH had undertaken to do this again. He used practically all of the available antibiotics now in use and for the first time he was able to demonstrate in our laboratory, as others have, strains resistant to tetracycline. They are also resistant to all the tetracyclines. The difference among the tetracyclines is as marked as I showed for other species —as much as 8 to 16-fold—for example with one of the new analogues, minocycline, as compared to tetracycline, but no antibiotics other than tetracyclines showed any change.

HOLT: To answer Prof. PULVERER's point, we published a letter last year in the Lancet explaining how we had found that about 10% of pneumococci in our hospital had become resistant to tetracycline, with an M.I.C. of perhaps 10 or 20 μg/ml. We also considered the possibility that only 1 or 2 serotypes were involved in this. In fact, we serotyped all the tetracycline-resistant strains and found a completely random distribution. We, like Dr. LUND, find many type 19's. We have never been able to understand this but we have always found a high percentage of type 19 strains. However, these are not necessarily more or less tetracycline-resistant than any other type.

FINLAND: A number of years ago we were confronted with an infection in our guinea pig colony that we were using for testing tubercle bacilli. For some reason or other, the bacteriologist, who was not acquainted with the literature on penicillin, injected every guinea-pig with 300,000 U of procaine penicillin and was amazed to find in the morning that all the guinea-pigs were dead. We knew this would happen from published work, but became interested in the bacteriology of the guinea-pig infection and found that this was a type 19 pneumococcus epidemic[1]. When we canvassed all of the guinea-pig colonies among animal growers or laboratories we found that type 19 pneumococcus was the prevalent strain throughout the United States and Canada. This was first demonstrated in Germany, as I recall. Now is that still the prevalent strain in the guinea-pig ?

LUND: Yes, when it is spontaneous infection, it is always type 19. They may be infected by other types but only experimentally.

[1] HOMBURGER, F., WILCOX, C., BARNES, M. W., FINLAND, M.: An epiziotic of pneumococcus type 19 infection in guinea pigs. Science **102**, 449—450 (1945)

II. Bacterial Infections:
Changes in their Causative Agents. Possible Reasons

Bayer-Symposium III, 62—67 (1971)

Non-Specific Mechanisms of Resistance to Infection and their Influence on the Changing Pattern of Causative Agents

E. H. Kass

The commonest sites of serious infection in hospitals today are in the broncho-pulmonary tree and in the urinary system. The mortality and morbidity rates from these infections continue to be high. Antimicrobial agents have had only limited usefulness in many of the clinical situations surrounding these groups of infections. In general, if one organism seems to be causing disease and is effectively eradicated and a second one replaces the first so that the underlying infectious process continues to progress, the problem can be solved in one of three ways. The first is to use a succession of drugs, which is what we generally have done. This has been of only modest benefit, as for example in the chronic bronchitic. Secondly, we may try to alter the available microbial flora to minimize the possibility of replacement. Thus we may try to free the gut of bacteria, or try to impose less pathogenic instead of more pathogenic organisms. Or we may take the longer term strategy of attempting to understand and perhaps thereby to influence host defenses, which must be a major variable influencing the ultimate outcome.

The present brief review will select a small number of aspects of the problem of host defenses, stressing the non-specific defenses in the lungs and in the urinary tract. Similar mechanisms in the gut will not be discussed at this time. Specific mechanisms will not be discussed. We are all aware that antibodies of different types are elaborated by or carried to the gut. It is still not clear how important these are in host defenses as major protective mechanisms in the gut, in the kidney, and in the bronchopulmonary tree.

The present review will discuss primarily those host defenses that do not seem to have a high level of specificity and that, as far as one can tell, account for the clearance of the majority of bacteria that are presented to these systems. In the pulmonary tree, leaving aside the air conditioning and filtering effect of the nasopharynx, one of the most important aspects of defense against microbes is that normally the lower bronchi and alveoli are sterile. This is so despite the continuous entry of bacteria to these areas. Traditionally this sterility has been thought to be due to the mucociliary apparatus of the bronchi. However if one thinks about this for a moment, an explanation based on the mucociliary apparatus could not possibly be adequate. In fact, we have been teaching, simultaneously, mutually contradictory ideas.

We agree on the one hand that when particles are in the range of 0.5 to 4.0 μ, they tend not to impinge on the bronchi but instead to remain suspended and be carried to the alveoli. This principle was worked out in relation to silicosis, but has been confirmed in innumerable ways. We also agree that bacterial aerosols, unless they are aggregated, or unless they are carried on squamous epithelium or things of this sort, form droplet nuclei that tend to be under 4 µ in diameter. From this it would follow that if we inhaled bacterial aerosols, they would not generally impinge on the bronchi. We are forced to the possibility that sterility in the lung could not be due exclusively to the function of the mucociliary apparatus.

For the past 8 or 10 years we have tested the implications of this point in our laboratory, with LAURENZI and BERMAN and later with GREEN and GOLDSTEIN, and now more recently with HUBER and LaForce. Much of the data has been collected in mice, some in rats, and occasionally in other animals. The present data will be limited to mice for the purpose of discussion, and we can talk of species variation when it is appropriate.

Mice are placed in an aerosol chamber, and the chamber is such that each mouse receives aerosols in which 85% of the particles are less than 4 µ in diameter. The mice are exposed for 30 min, and the bacterial count in the aerosol is regulated so that about 50,000 colonies will be cultivated from the homogenized lungs of the mice at the end of the 30 min exposure. Immediately after such an exposure, a rapid decline in the number of viable bacteria in the lungs occurs, so that at 4 h about 85% of a strain of *S. aureus* will have been removed. In 6 h, about 92% of the staphylococci are gone. This disappearance or clearance differs for different microorganisms, which argues against the importance of the mucociliary apparatus, since the different bacterial species are approximately the same size and yet *Staphylococcus albus* is cleared more rapidly than *S. aureus* and *S. aureus* is cleared more rapidly than a strain of *P. mirabilis* that happened to be used in these experiments. If this disappearance is, as suggested, due principally to killing *in situ* in the lung rather than to mechanical transport from the lung by the mucociliary apparatus, it should be possible to test the hypothesis quite precisely by the use of radiolabeled bacteria.

The argument is a simple one. If the bacteria are radiolabeled (in this case with P_{32}) and if the removal of bacteria is due to mechanical transport, then the labels should be removed simultaneously with loss of viability. If, on the other hand, the bacteria are killed in the lung, then the labels should remain after the bacteria are nonviable, and that is what happens. Only about 15 to 20% of the disappearance of bacteria from the lung can possibly be due to transport. The remainder represents *in situ* killing. Bacteria and bacterial cell wall antigens can be found within the alveolar macrophages of the animal's lungs. Thus there is an extremely potent antibacterial system throughout the lung.

Next we explored this active system in detail to study some clinically applicable situations in which the clearance of bacteria may be affected by environmental conditions.

Two aspects of this are particularly interesting. The first is that environmental circumstances affect the clearance of bacteria strikingly. Secondly, the phagocytosis of different bacteria is affected differently by the same environmental conditions. For example, the clearance of staphylococci (whether *S. aureus* or *S. albus*) is significantly depressed by ethyl alcohol, and the depression is linear with dose of alcohol. In the case of Proteus, this is not only true, but also

Proteus will multiply in the lungs of animals given sufficient doses of ethanol, leading to pneumonia. In a few moments, I will also tell you about the depressant effects of cigarette smoke. We did not investigate all of the pleasures of man.

The next environmental condition that will be discussed for this purpose is hypoxia. A simulated 10,000 foot altitude is less likely to affect clearance of Proteus than it is to affect the clearance of staphylococci, whereas with ethanol, there is a much greater effect on the Proteus system, permitting multiplication. Immersion of the animals into cold water, corticosteroids, starvation, and acidosis inhibit bacterial clearance by the murine lung. Male animals and female animals differ quite significantly in their relative susceptibility to such environmental stimuli as ethanol and hypoxia; the male is much more affected by ethanol than is the female.

An experiment that is of particular interest has to do with candidiasis in the mouse. When Candida are injected into the mouse, the organisms appear in the lung and disappear slowly, and appear in the kidney but multiply in the latter organ, and the animals ultimately die of advanced renal failure. The bacterial clearance is not affected until the animals have become azotemic. Nephrectomy produces a similar effect. In some manner, acidosis and azotemia depress bacterial clearance by the lung.

The use of radioactive phosphate to label bacteria can be so precise that it is possible to use one animal as his own control. If one knows the ratio of label to viability in the initial aerosol, one can kill the animal at 4 or 6 h and from the viability and the total amount of radioactivity in the lung at the latter point, one can estimate the percentage of the original inoculum that was killed by the lung. This becomes a sensitive and efficient technique for studying bacterial clearance.

Another interesting effect is seen in the bacterial-virus interaction. When influenza virus infection is produced in the mouse using a sublethal dose of PR8 strain, and the animals then are exposed to bacteria, the initial bacterial clearance is quite normal. Clearance remains normal until some time between the 6th and 9th day when clearance becomes markedly depressed, after which the depressed clearance disappears. The same effect has been observed with repiratory syncytial virus, an organism that multiplies little in the lung. This effect is interesting clinically because in general when bacterial pneumonias are superimposed on viral respiratory illness, they often occur about 1 week after the initial respiratory episode.

Cigarette smoke is an unusually powerful source of inhibition of the pulmonary macrophage mechanisms. GREEN and CAROLIN studied macrophages harvested from bronchi of rabbits, and found that when a cigarette was "smoked" by withdrawal into a syringe, as little as 2 ml of the smoke significantly inhibited the capacity of the macrophages to kill staphylococci. The material in the cigarette smoke that does this is not yet known. It is labile and the effect is overcome by glutathione and other sulfahydryl compounds.

Recently, HUBER and associates have shown that ozone in the atmosphere in concentrations of under one part per million had a similar depressant effect on the capacity of the lungs to clear bacteria. Since ozone is a powerful oxidant, attention turned to oxygen alone, and it was found that oxygen supplied to the animal in concentrations above ambient concentrations were depressive to the macrophages. The oxygen effect is reversible and is accompanied by ultrastructural and phospholipid changes in the macrophage that seem quite characteristic.

Some possible clinical relationships may be suggested by these observations. For example, if animals are exposed to a Staphylococcus and Proteus, the two species are cleared at normal rates, that is, the capacity of the lung to clear these bacteria is so large that the presentation of both organisms at the same time does not influence the rate of clearance of either. This effect can be observed by labelling the two organisms with different radioactive labels. Now, if the animals are placed in an hypoxic environment and exposed to a mixture of the two organisms, the clearance of Proteus is not affected by hypoxia but the clearance of Staphylococcus is depressed. At one point, the Proteus may have been removed and the Staphylococcus still remained, so that at the right moment one may find a pure culture of Staphylococcus, with no Proteus remaining. Conversely, if a mixture of the two species of bacteria is administered to animals given alcohol, the staphylococci are removed and the Proteus remains. So one can get a pure culture from the mixture just by manipulation of the environment. This suggests some relevance to what we see in more complex disease states.

We know little about the pulmonary macrophage system. We don't know whether it represents a discrete cell type or several types of cells. The cells that have been washed out of the bronchi have received most of the study, and these may represent wandering systemic macrophages as well as those that have broken away from the alveoli. The attached cells of the alveoli may have quite different metabolic properties. There is an important anatomical problem which has not yet been solved, but is being actively pursued.

Metabolically, the pulmonary macrophages that are washed out of the bronchi differ from peritoneal macrophages in a number of ways, but the significance of the differences is not known. Peritoneal macrophages are less susceptible to anaerobiasis than are pulmonary macrophages and have corresponding differences in cytochrome. It is not known whether this is adaptive or is intrinsic in the cell line. Lysosome content, various phosphatase activities, and lactic dehydrogenase activities are different in pulmonary and peritoneal macrophages, but again we do not know whether this is intrinsic in the cell line or adaptive to the specific circumstances of the lung.

This may be a good point at which to stop and to move to the urinary tract, as the other area in which we can discuss non-specific mechanisms. In the urinary tract, the non-specific defence mechanisms are quite different from those in the lung. The empirical observation that provides a basis for attack of the problem is first that the bacterial content of the urethra is greatest near the external meatus and decreases proximally. Secondly, when bacteria are put into the bladder in experimental animals, there is often spontaneous disappearance of the bacteria. In the human being, there is often a spontaneous loss of bacteriuria. It is difficult to explain this spontaneous loss of bacteriuria. Most people do not void frequently enough or have sufficient diuresis to account for disappearance of the bacteria on a simple dilutional basis. In general, many bacteria find urine to be an excellent culture medium. The bacteria are increasing geometrically, and the addition of new urine provides only arithmetic dilution. Therefore if bacteria are to be eliminated from the bladder under conditions in which there is not enforced diuresis, it is necessary to postulate some type of antibacterial action in the bladder that slows bacterial multiplication.

If bladder homogenates are examined for an effect that is inhibitory to *E. coli*, no evidence of such an activity is found. If, however, a flap of viable bladder mucosa is inoculated with tiny volumes of a bacterial culture, the bacteria are killed rapidly and 90 to 99% are killed within a brief time. That this is killing and not washing off by exudate is shown by experiments with radiolabelled bacteria. In these experiments, there is convincing evidence that the bacteria are killed on the surface of the bladder. In similar experiments, labelled bacteria have been applied to the urethral surface, and a similar local killing effect was demonstrable.

These experiments are admittedly artificial. It was desirable to study bacterial killing in the unmanipulated bladder. In such experiments, the following line of reasoning was followed. If bacteria are labeled with a radiolabel and there is a known ratio between the bacterial count and the radiolabel, then if there is killing of the bacteria *in situ*, the label will remain but the bacterial count will decline. If, on the other hand, the animal discharges the urine without killing bacteria, the ratio would be unchanged but the total number of viable bacterial units and the total amount of radioactivity will decline. If there is both voiding and killing, the total amount of viability and radioactivity will decline but the ratio will change to the degree that killing has occurred. So it is possible in this system to study dynamically what happens in the bladder and measure killing accurately while measuring the effect of voiding. Experiments with this system show that the bladder of the guinea pig and of the rat kills bacteria rapidly *in situ*. Curiously, *E. coli* is killed more rapidly than *S. aureus*, and we don't know what this means or whether it is peculiar to the guinea pig, in which these experiments were conducted.

An alternative explanation for these data is that there is not killing but that there is simply bacterial clumping. And if the bacteria aggregate so that there are ten bacteria at one locus instead of one, then this would also give a decline in the number of apparent viable units without a change in radioactivity. This possibility was tested by examining serial sections of the bladder. Whenever bacteria were found, they were individual and not clumped so that the clumping explanation does not seem to be sufficient.

Thus, there is an antibacterial activity in the mucosa of the bladder. We haven't a clear statement of what this consists of except that it happens too rapidly to be due to polymorphonuclear leukocytes or other exudate components. Our working hypothesis at the moment is that the killing effect is due to the release of metabolic acid from the mucosa, and the metabolic acid inhibits bacteria that are closely applied to the mucosa. At the right pH, metabolic acids rapidly inhibit bacteria. This general explanation is attractive because it would help to explain the clinical situations in which a residual pool of urine left in the bladder is associated with persistence of bacteriuria without bacterial killing. Bacteria must be directly against the mucosa for killing to occur so that if there is an indwelling catheter or if there is obstruction, the bladder cannot completely empty and the bacteria are not cleared spontaneously but will persist.

In the kidney, in contrast to the bladder, there are several mechanisms that affect resistance to bacterial multiplication. It is now well demonstrated that it is the medulla of the kidney and not the cortex that is the preferred site of bacterial multiplication. The radiation to the cortex is secondary to the bacterial multiplication in the medulla. The increased susceptibility of the medulla is related in some way to the blood flow and to the osmolality of medulla. The medulla has about one-tenth the blood flow and higher osmolality than does the cortex. This can be tested experimentally. For example, one can produce hemorrhagic hypotension to reduce the blood flow to the cortex to the same levels that occur in the medulla, and under those conditions bacteria injected into the cortex multiply just as they do in the medulla. Also, FEKETY and ROCHA produced burns in the kidney at different levels with a microcautery. The rate at which inflammation appeared in the medulla was several hours slower than the rate at which inflammation appeared in the cortex, and presumably this is an important basis whereby bacteria multiply in the medulla preferentially. In addition, high concentrations of various solutes such as urea and salts, which may occur in the papilla, inhibit to some degree phagocytosis by phagocytic cells. Finally, BEESON and ROWLEY have shown that enough ammonia may be manufactured in the medulla to inhibit the fourth component of complement and therefore to interfere with both phagocytic and killing processes. Diuresis reduces the osmolality of the medulla and is associated with decreased bacterial multiplication in the medulla.

I have tried to indicate that protection against bacteria has evolved in different ways for the lung and the urinary tract. Parenthetically, protective mechanisms in the gut differ from those of the other two systems.

Thus, there are powerful, relatively non-selective mechanisms that are likely to be quite susceptible to environmental circumstances and to internal metabolic changes. Surely these must play a role in our consideration of the problem of reduced resistance in clinical infection. One of our tasks is to determine how to manipulate these understandings in order to control the clinical situation.

Prof. E. H. KASS
Director
Channing Laboratory
Professor of Medicine
Harvard Medical School
City of Boston Department Health and Hospitals
818 Harrison Avenue
Boston (Massachusetts) 02118, U.S.A.

Discussion

GSELL: I have two questions to ask. What are the possibilities that the response of the lung is nonspecific? Could you do the same thing not only with young mice but also with older ones? Perhaps then there would be some change. Perhaps the same would be true if you repeat these exposures—with smoke, for example. Is there always the same response or is their a change in response?

KASS: These are interesting questions. This can be studied in rats as GARETH GREEN has done. Older rats develop bronchitis spontaneously. The bronchitic rat, in general, clears bacteria very much like the younger rat but there are always a few animals who clear the bacteria much more slowly. If one examines a pathogen such as *Pasteurella pneumoseptica* in mice, an organism which produces a fatal infection, the majority of the inhaled bacteria are eliminated exactly as are staphylococci or *Proteus* but there are always a few mice that depart from the normal distribution curve and eliminate the bacteria very slowly. The pathogenicity rests in that few.

This may be like the phenomenon that Prof. REBER was talking about. The majority of animals handle the pathogen very well but a few can not eliminate the pathogen efficiently. This is curious and interesting. It makes this type of situation realistic as a model but this is all we know.

MARGET: Have you any experience in comparing animals with and without antibiotics in this experiment?

KASS: We have not used any antibiotics in our experiments. I also meant to respond to one other point raised by Prof. GSELL. We have performed repeated exposures to staphylococci daily and the curve is always the same: repeated exposures seem not to saturate the system. I think the reason is that the system is so huge in its potential that repeated exposures of the size we use do not do very much to inhibit the system.

The capacity of the alveolar macrophage system is seen in another experiment performed by GOLDSTEIN. When he produced silicosis in the mouse it had very little effect on bacterial clearance except when the animals become acidotic, because earlier, even though the lungs were solidly involved with silicosis, the changes were still focal and there was enough potential left in the remainder of the lung to take care of the inhaled bacteria. The anatomical lesion itself was not as important as the general metabolic one which affected all of the cells.

GSELL: In silicosis in man where, during many years, nothing happens, perhaps the response of the other part of the lung is very good.

KASS: This fits the clinical situation in man in which in early silicosis, there is little if any trouble, and the trouble comes only when respiratory failure occurs. It would be nice if someone could think of a way to study this type of clearance in the intact human being.

PULVERER: What do you mean by sterile? Do you mean also anaerobically sterile? I ask this because we found that in the lower and upper bronchi there are normally anaerobes from the mucosa of the mouth.

KASS: One can find, down to a few inches below the carina, any of the organisms that might be found in the oropharynx or in the gastrointestinal tract. Basically, the respiratory and gastrointestinal tracts are a continuum. The same organisms are found in both places but their distribution differs. However below the primary bronchi, in the normal individual, neither anaerobes nor aerobes can be cultured.

DASCHNER: Dr. KASS, what do you think is the clinical significance of the clearance of bacteria from the bladder mucosa in rats? You postulate a direct contact of the bacteria with the mucosa but most of the bacteria in the urine are not in contact with bladder mucosa in the course of the infection.

KASS: It gets down to how big a volume of urine is left lining the mucosa after complete voiding. I cannot give any quantitative figure but we have guessed that from 0.1 to 2 ml could be still lining the mucosa in a very thin layer without forming a pool after micturition. Under those conditions we can expect the antibacterial mechanism to be operating. If the pool of urine gets any larger, then the mechanism could not possibly operate. The question gets down to what amount of urine one thinks is still left in the bladder after voiding.

MARGET: Did you do the clearance study of bacteria in man?

KASS: We have, and so have HINMAN and Cox. We all have seen clinically the spontaneous clearance of bacteriuria at variable periods of time—over a few days to many days.

MARGET: Have you done pre-treatment with endotoxin in the bladder?

KASS: We did a series of experiments with endotoxin and have seen no change in clearance. However, the amounts of endotoxin were very small; they were calculated to produce no effect on the body temperature of the animal and it may be that they were too small to produce any effect. We want to go back to these experiments.

BARTMANN: Just one question. Is the clearance of bacteria from the bladder dependent on the pH of the urine?

KASS: In a general way the answer is No; that is, one can get the same clearance of bacteria in the rabbit, which has an alkaline urine, and in the rat which has an acid urine. I believe, but cannot yet prove it, that the critical fact, namely, the metabolic acid production at the surface, is probably so great that the local environment is what matters. As soon as that local effect is diluted, the urinary pH is so much higher that it would probably not matter very much. This is based on the hypothesis that the unionized molecules of organic acid are the lethal agents and that the pH of the urine would seldom be low enough to affect favourably the local killing action.

Bayer-Symposium III, 71—76 (1971)
© by Springer-Verlag 1971

Opportunists and Opportunity in Infection

J. C. GOULD

There is an increasing awareness of certain changes in the nature of infection occurring in hospital, particularly in the type of microflora which is predominant in such infections. Most notably gram-negative bacilli as causes of infection have excited comment in recent years and other groups of organisms have become more common.

The opportunities for infection in the past have been largely provided by ignorance of the germ theory of disease, the lack of hygiene and medical and nursing discipline, and the subjection of patients to procedures which short circuit the normal defence mechanisms. In the past this undoubtedly contributed to a high incidence of infection and whilst such causes are involved to a much lesser extent to-day there are further factors which contribute to infection and to the nature of the organisms which cause it.

The opportunists in the past included multitudes of pathogens and potential pathogens, many the cause of epidemic disease such as dysentery, typhoid, cholera, gas gangrene and the many forms of pyogenic infection. Most of these infections, particularly bacterial infections, have been very successfully controlled and perhaps this has been largely lost sight of during the emphasis given to such problems of infection that have continued in recent years. The reduction in morbidity is not as striking as the reduction in mortality, but most epidemic infections have been controlled or have disappeared, and most acute infections are aborted before patients are considered for admission to hospital. Thus the pattern of infection in hospital has changed radically from the period before antibiotics were available. It is this change in the pattern of disease with which we are at present concerned and this is associated with a marked ecological change in the causative microflora and the greater importance of species not normally regarded as pathogenic to man.

Is this a straight forward process of change resulting from more living room for those organisms which previously could not compete with the more virulent pathogens now controlled by antimicrobial agents ? The alteration of the environment by selective factors such as antibiotics and antiseptics has undoubtedly eliminated many species and has allowed the spread of varieties which are resistant to these agents. This is particularly important in relation to the emergence and propagation of specifically resistant bacteria.

Thus our opportunists at the present time consist of a) organisms that are antibiotic resistant variants of normally sensitive species such as *Staphylococcus* and *Escherichia*, b) organisms which are basically antibiotic resistant and which may be pathogenic such as *Monilia*, and c) organisms which are either sapro- phytic or of low pathogenicity and which for various reasons find themselves in a situation in which they are able to produce infection either by themselves or associated with other microflora, e.g. *Pseudomonas*, *Achromobacter* and *Serratia*.

These micro-organisms are all favoured by an environment which is made selective by factors which allow them to survive while being in some way unsuitable to other microflora. In such a selective environment the opportunities for infection may be provided by variation in the following factors:

1. Apparatus and Instruments Used

The efficiency of sterilisation procedures such as autoclaving may be reduced and allow organisms to be introduced into fluids and on instruments and lead to infection. Other forms of apparatus such as respirators, anaesthetic machines, humidifiers and baths, present great hazards if they are not properly maintained and cleansed.

2. The Procedures Which are Used to Treat Patients

The dangers inherent in many types of procedure used in treatment should be fully recognised. Such procedures may be relatively simple such as venipuncture and catheterisation; others may be complicated, such as transfusion, cardiac catheterisation or prolonged and difficult surgical operations. Not only do such procedures carry with them the risk of direct introduction of micro-organisms but they are often associated with other forms of treatment which specifically reduce the patient's resistance to infection.

3. Environmental Factors

The environment of the patient may be modified in various ways. The selective effect of antibiotics, antiseptics and other chemotherapeutic agents has already been referred to and the use of such substances must be intelligently controlled to avoid the unnecessary selection of resistant flora. Where necessary the patient with reduced resistance to infection or subject to hazardous procedures should be protected from unnecessary hazards of infection in the environment and to this end the use of isolation facilities in hospitals is often necessary.

4. The Patient

The normal physical defence mechanisms of the patient may be breeched by introducing instruments which if contaminated will introduce organisms into the tissues. Commensal flora may be upset or removed by over-enthusiastic use of antimicrobial agents and thus further diminish the patients defences. The immunity of the patient may be lowered by the use of radiation or drugs for the purposes of transplantation or the treatment of neoplastic disease and additional care is very necessary to prevent infection. The following are some examples of the more common situations in which opportunistic organisms may procedure infection.

Respiratory Tract

Invasion of the respiratory tract by organisms of low pathogenicity is not a rare occurrence and cases with extensive invasion by *Candida albicans* have been reported. *Aspergillus* species may sometimes invade the lung and rapidly progressive disease may be associated with such other opportunistic bacteria as, e.g. *Pseudomonas pyocyanea* (KENNEDY, MALONE and BLYTH, 1970). More common is the isolation of antibiotic-resistant gram-negative bacilli from the upper respiratory tract secretions and sputa of patients with chronic bronchitis and other pulmonary infections who are under antibiotic treatment (Table 1). Less common is invasion of the lung tissues by these organisms. The hazard to the patient from these organisms, however, must be increased by the conditions which allow their colonisation. The most important of these are long term chemotherapy and being in hospital (Table 1).

The prevention of colonisation and possible tissue invasion by these opportunistic organisms depends upon the treatment of susceptible patients who require

Table 1. *Colonisation of the respiratory tract by antibiotic-resistant coliform bacilli*

	Proportion of patients colonised %	Proportion of colonised patients requiring specific treatment %
Long-stay patients in neurological department	90	35
Chronic bronchitis in respiratory disease department	40	10
Out-patients	<10	1

hospitalisation in strict isolation so as to avoid contamination with hospital micro-organisms which may be antibiotic resistant. If the patient can be treated at home this is a better solution. In all such patients antimicrobial agents should be prescribed with circumspection to avoid unnecessary upset of the commensal flora and proliferation of abnormal species.

Intestinal Tract

Infections of the gut may be produced by organisms of low pathogenicity and this is more likely if there is interference of the normal commensal flora.

It is common practice in many hospitals to use antibiotic and other antimicrobial drugs for the preparation of the bowel prior to operation. Many of these drugs are used orally because of their relatively poor absorption from the gut, e.g. the aminoglycosides, but it is generally believed that oral antibiotics carry a greater risk of upsetting the commensal microflora and subsequent superinfection with abnormal flora which is antibiotic resistant, e.g. *Staphylococcus* or *Candida*. An increase in resistant organisms with low pathogenicity, particularly *Klebsiella*, *Pseudomonas* and *Proteus*, does also undoubtedly occur following antibiotic treatment, particularly if this is prolonged (Table 2).

The population of the lower bowel is high and consists predominantly of strict anaerobes which are found in greater numbers when the flow of gut contents is slow (Table 3). The micro-aerophilic flora which includes *Escherichia* and *Streptococcus*, is very much the minority comprising normally less than 1% of the total

Table 2. *Colonisation of lower bowel with opportunist organisms. Numbers of Pseudomonas, Klebsiella, Proteus and Monilia isolated, per gram of faeces*

On admission to hospital	After limited chemotherapy	After 6 weeks in hospital without chemotherapy	After prolonged chemotherapy
$10-10^3$	10^2-10^5	10^2-10^5	10^3-10^7

Table 3. *Normal faecal flora*

	Viable counts/Gm
Microaerophilic organisms	
Escherichia coli	10^7
Streptococcus	10^6
Lactobacilli	10^5
Staphylococcus	10^3
Bacillus	10^2
Yeasts	10^2
Anaerobes	
Lactobacillus bifidus	10^{9-12}
Bacteroides	10^{8-11}
Clostridium	10^{5-6}

microflora. It is however this flora which is first affected by antibacterial substances in the gut. Most persons carry small numbers of other micro-aerophilic species in the lumen of the bowel and such organisms will increase in number during antibiotic treatment at the expense of the normal flora. The anaerobic micro-organisms, however, are more slowly reduced by antibacterial agents, unless there is flux, and it appears that as long as they are maintained, large increases in the number of abnormal microaerophilic bacteria are prevented (Table 3). To this end short courses of antibiotics are preferable.

Infection in Neonates and Children

The environment, particularly in hospital, may contain antibiotic-resistant saprophytes such as *Serratia* and *Pseudomonas* and these may contaminate patients as a result of various procedures and the use of contaminated instruments. Once established in the tissues these organisms may be difficult to eradicate. Patients with reduced defence mechanisms are peculiarly liable to infections with such organisms as also is the new born child. Reservoirs of these saprophytic opportunists are incubators and respirators, "sterile" water supplies in wards and surgical theatres, and contamination from such sources may lead to infection. These infections are more common in premature infants and those with congenital abnormality but can also occur in normal infants. In cases of spina bifida, bacteremia and meningitis may occur and the introduction of contaminated water or the use of instruments which have been stored in infected antiseptics may lead to wound sepsis, or, after bladder irrigation, cystitis. The establishment of *Pseudomonas* in the intestinal tract may produce enteritis, and on the skin, necrotic pustular lesions. The eyes may be infected, resulting in severe conjunctivitis.

The prevention of such infections depends upon ensuring that apparatus is free of contamination with these opportunist organisms and that antiseptic substances used to cleanse apparatus and instruments is itself not contaminated with, and supporting the growth of such organisms. The antibiotics which are used in the treatment of the patient should not act in a selective manner to encourage the spread of these resistant opportunists and when specific treatment is required, care should be taken to select a drug or combination of drugs which is specifically effective against the causative organism.

Summary

Conditions similar to those which encourage the selection and spread of antibiotic resistant variants of pathogenic species increase the possibility of infection due to organisms of low pathogenicity and these are the opportunists of the present day. These conditions include the use of antibiotics and other antimocrobial agents both in the general and micro environment of the patient, which act as powerful selective factors. Opportunists tend to be organisms having a high resistance to most of the antibacterial agents in common use.

Other conditions which are necessary for organisms of low pathogenicity to establish themselves include the use of contaminated apparatus, procedures carried out in patients which are conducive to the spread of these organisms and patients who are in a state of diminished resistance owing to intercurrent illness, congenital abnormalities or specific interference with their natural defence mechanisms.

To reduce the hazard of infection with antibiotic resistant organisms and opportunists, restriction in the use of antimicrobial agents is required so that undue ecological pressures due to their presence are not produced. Further, the greatest care is required in the cleaning and maintenance of apparatus used in the treatment and management of patients; in disinfection and sterilisation, and in carrying out procedures which involve interference with the patient and his normal defence mechanisms.

Reference

Kennedy, W. P. U., Malone, D. N., Blyth, W.: Thorax 25, 691 (1970).

Dr. J. C. Gould
South-Eastern Regional Hospital Board
Central Microbiological Laboratories
Western General Hospital
Crewe Road
Edinburgh, EH4 2XU (Scotland)

Discussion

Reber: This notion of "opportunists" is a very interesting one, but is this new notion necessary? This notion emerges as an essential part of microbial life; every microbe is an opportunist. For example, the polio virus previously caused one case of real disease among every 100 to 200 infections; the diphtheria bacillus causes disease only ten times out of 200 infections. These are opportunists because of the susceptibility of the host. Opportunism is a real property of every parasite; it is a property of life. We are all opportunists; we cannot survive without opportunism, without a use of the conditions given by our environment. So that this notion of opportunist is not a new one.

Naumann: I have one question concerning Dr. Gould's results on the increase of *Pseudomonas*, *Candida* and other saprophytic strains in faeces under therapy. Did you find any differences depending on the route of administration, that is, any differences between the oral and the parenteral route?

Gould: I am not really able to answer that question myself because the great majority of the cases that I have referred to in these figures were treated by the oral route.

Kass: With respect to the important point that relates to anaerobic flora in the gut, we should recall that the multiplication rates of many anaerobes are different from those of coliforms. *Bacteriodes*, with a generation time of many hours, may not compete successfully with *E. coli* or *Proteus* which have generation times of 15 or 20 min. Therefore, even though *Bacteriodes* may outnumber the facultative organisms in the gut by 2 or 3 logs, they will be rapidly outnumbered by the coliforms in the usual culture medium, and this may be quite relevant to what happens in exudates and other body fluids.

Gould: I would answer Dr. Kass by asking him "Does he not think that under suitable conditions the oxidation-reduction potential in the lumen of the gut at the normal speed of passage is more suitable for the more rapid growth of anaerobic species such as *Bacteriodes* and even of *Lactobacillus*, their multiplication matches that of *Escherichia coli*.

Kass: No, under suitable anaerobic conditions (e.g. 100 to 125 mv) it still takes 3 or 4 days for full growth of most strains of *Bacteriodes*.

GOULD: I think if one goes to a very much lower Eh than 120 or even 380 to 400 mv and less, it is then that you find that the generation time of *Bacteriodes* is very much less. This is certainly so in the condition obtainable in the laboratory model.

FINLAND: I would like to recall to you a study that was done by Dr. GABUZDA and several others of my associates on the aerobic bacterial flora during the administration of antibiotics to essentially normal—but somewhat under-nourished—adult males[1].

We did total counts and counts of specific species and essentially confirmed what you said, Dr. GOULD. But the interesting thing about the administration of antibiotics is that the early result, as far as aerobes are concerned, is the very marked and drastic reduction in the number of aerobes, both gram-negative and gram-positive organisms—with some increase in *Candida* if that organism was part of the basic flora. The increase in *Candida* is slow but our observations extended to 9 days of control and 9 days of treatment, first with absorbable antibiotics like tetracycline, then with non-absorbable ones like the combination of polymyxin and bacitracin. In every instance, during the antibiotic period, there was initially a marked reduction of between 7 and 8 logs in the number of bacteria per gram of faeces but in the rebound, when there was regrowth by the end of 9 days, we often had 10^{11} to 10^{12} organisms/g of faeces. In other words, we had practically a solid bacterial mass. This is an interesting feature of the continued administration of antibiotics and is also true even with the non-absorbable antibiotics.

GOULD: Are you referring to 10^{12} anaerobes or aerobes per gram?

FINLAND: We did not consider the anaerobic flora at all; this is merely a reflection of the aerobic flora that we were culturing during the administration of the antibiotics.

GOULD: I have never encountered such large numbers of aerobes in faeces. Were these patients who had diarrhoea—or a flux after antibiotic therapy—or those who had constipation?

FINLAND: No, these were people—and we had pictures of their faecal output during the various periods—control and drug administration. What happened was that the bulk of their faeces increased very much and they had a feeling of fullness, but they did not have diarrhoea; they may have had loose stools because they have a more frequent urge to get rid of these large masses of soft, light faeces.

ERICSSON: Let us leave the observations which Dr. GOULD presented and also the discussion; where it is obvious that you do not influence the anaerobes—you do not influence the opportunists and after some time you stimulate the aerobes. My question is: "Why should antibiotics, in any situation which I could think of, but mainly prophylactically, before bowel surgery, be used at all? Is not the

---

[1] GABUZDA, G. J., GOCKE, J. M., JACKSON, G. G., GRIGSBY, M. E., DEL LOVE, B.: Some effects of antibiotics on malnutrition in man, including studies of the antibacterial flora of the feces. Arch. intern. Med. 101, 476—513 (1958).

biologically sound answer to the biological dilemma here, to rotate the antibiotics, not to use them at all prophylactically but to use them selectively, and monitoring the results so that you know what bacteria you are fighting and what you are really aiming at? I have the same attitude to the prophylactic use of antibiotics as any priest has to sin! I am against it!

GOULD: My suggestion of a restrictive and rotational policy in the hospital's use of antibiotics was not intended to refer to the prophylactic use of antibiotics nor in surgery of the bowel, I was using the data on the effect of oral antibiotics on the intestinal flora merely as an illustration of the mechanism of opportunistic infection or superinfection leading to such conditions as enterocolitis. My conclusions were that if the antibiotics are used only for a short time and changed from patient to patient, there is less possibility of a harmful effect, as there is less effect upon the anaerobic flora of the intestinal tract. Under such conditions this residual commensal flora has greater difficulty in multiplying and establishing itself.

My general implication was that in the treatment of infections in closed surgical or medical units, that perhaps there is some benefit from imposing some sort of restrictive policy other than that which we have been using up to now. Certainly our local experience indicates that some benefit is derived from the use of single—or a limited number of agents which one changes periodically, as judged by a progressive fall in infection rates and mortality.

FINLAND: I would like to mention one situation in which we have been using oral antibiotics, which is indigenous to the Boston City Hospital, but I understand is also not infrequent in other parts of the world. We have a large number of alcoholics and some of them take enough alcohol to destroy their liver and they come to us with liver failure. It has been shown by Dr. CHARLES LIEBER and others, and before that by Dr. BAIRD HASTINGS and his associates, and as a matter of fact, even earlier by Dr. CHARLES S. DAVIDSON, that the liberation of ammonia into the blood stream is at least associated with liver failure and coma. HASTINGS and LIEBER showed that this was related to the production of ammonia in the bowel by *E. coli*—or some coliforms—but particularly *E. coli*, and this ammonia production was inhibited by the use of antibiotics. Dr. LIEBER showed that with tetracycline, but neomycin also does the same and perhaps even better, because it is not absorbed. In respect to anaerobes, it is interesting that neomycin, like all other aminoglycosides, does not affect the anaerobic gram-negatives so that we are specifically acting on the aerobic organism and the ammonia producing flora.

SHOOTER: I would like to say something about prophylactic chemotherapy. Some years ago Prof. WILLIAMS and I, working together in our open wards, observed patients—30% of whom would come in carrying staphylococci and during their stay their rate of carriage rose to about 70%. This, we felt—although not everyone agreed with us—was dangerous because the strains they picked up tended to be hospital strains, some of them associated with high incidences of infections. But in another ward where the patients were in much smaller units, they came in with about the same rate of carriers and during their stay the rate dropped. This was a chest service where prophylactic chemotherapy was used and where the sepsis rate was low. Prophylactic chemotherapy in this sort of circumstance, where you are not getting transmission of staphylococcal hospital infection, should not be compared directly with chemotherapy in situations in which there is a high rate of nasal staphylococci.

FINLAND: If Prof. WILLIAMS is going to tell us to use prophylaxis tomorrow, then I think we are all going to have a good argument.

SHOOTER: I think you have to look carefully and examine the situations in which prophylactic chemotherapy are used.

FINLAND: No doubt there is a lot of food for thought and a lot of basis for additional experiments along the lines of the changing pattern of bacteria. Does anybody have any specific questions? (No questions!).

Bayer-Symposium III, 81—87 (1971)
© by Springer-Verlag 1971

The Colonisation of Ventriculo-Atrial Shunts by Coagulase-Negative Staphylococci

R. J. HOLT

With 5 Figures

Several workers have reported to this Syposium studies on virulent bacterial pathogens well known to cause severe infection; at the other end of the scale, and in complete contrast, the present paper describes investigations on an indolent condition so low-grade that clinical symptoms frequently remain undetected for many months, and which is now regarded by many authorities as an example of colonisation rather than infection.

The past decade has seen the increasing use of artificial internal prostheses for the repair of cardiac defects, for the replacement of defective heart valves, and for the drainage of excess fluid from the cerebral ventricles, and in each case it is common experience that a very considerable proportion of these prostheses will eventually become colonised by bacteria, with an accompanying bacteraemia. At Queen Mary's Hospital about 100 ventriculo-atrial shunts are inserted each year into the cerebral ventricles of very young babies for the relief of hydrocephalus, draining excess fluid directly into the right atrium of the heart (Fig. 1) or indirectly into the azygos vein; they may also drain into body cavities, and are usually implanted in the first 3 weeks of life. The shunt is operative for the first 5 to 7 years of life, after which it is hoped that the hydrocephalus will spontaneously arrest and the shunt can be removed; the distal catheter must be lengthened once or twice during this period to compensate for natural growth.

During these years it seems certain that some 10 to 12% of these shunts will become colonised with bacteria and that these bacteria will also appear in the bloodstream. The detection of bacteraemia is almost always the first sign of colonisation, which may manifest itself only after many months or years of successful function, with little or no leucocyte response in the ventricles or the blood. What is surprising is that this colonisation is almost invariably caused by coagulase-negative staphylococci. Only four exceptions to this have been seen in the past 10 years at Queen Mary's in well over 100 separate incidents of shunt colonisation: two were caused by Candida, one by an enterococcus and, very recently, one by a diphtheroid which had colonised the shunt lumen. The last case was atypical in that the shunt was inserted soon after birth to drain a subdural haematoma but was judged to have ceased functioning after 1 year and had remained *in situ* for a further 3 years.

The further classification of coagulase-negative staphylococci has long presented many problems; quite recently two distinct schemes have become available, a biotyping system devised by BAIRD-PARKER (1963) and experimental phage typing schemes developed by Prof. R. E. O. Williams in London and Prof. Winkler and his colleagues in Utrecht. The biotyping system revealed that the shunt colonising strains at Queen Mary's and several other hospitals in the United Kingdom always belonged to the Baird-Parker subgroup S.II, a subgroup common on child and adult skin, in and outside hospital, but by no means exclusively so.

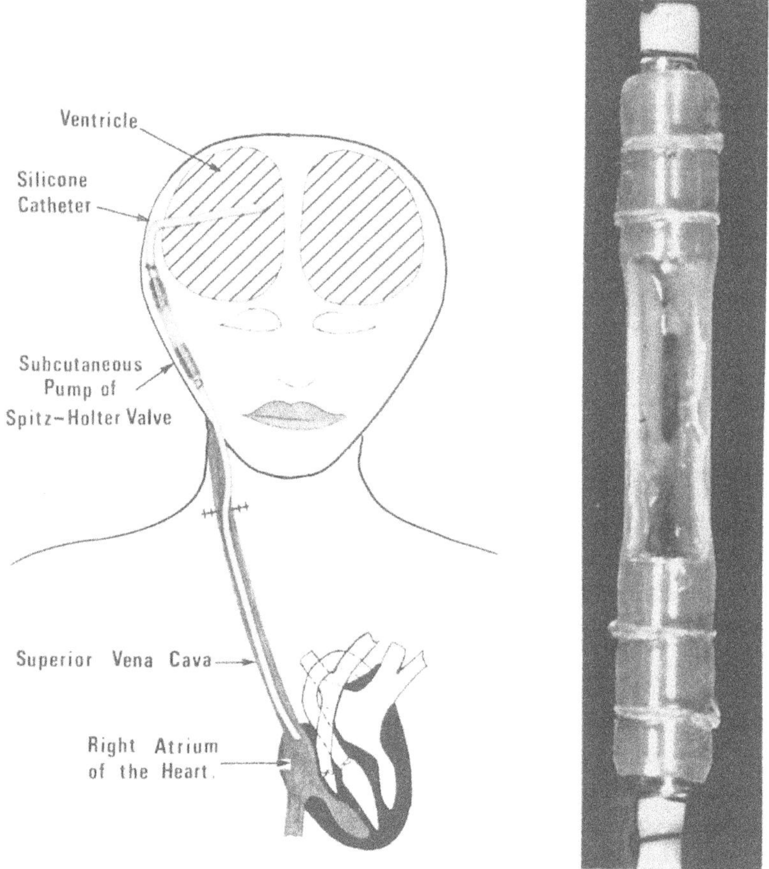

Fig. 1   Fig.2

Fig. 1. *Ventriculo-atrial shunt* with *Spitz-Holter valve* for drainage of excess fluid from cerebral ventricles

Fig. 2. *Lumen of valve* from ventriculo-atrial shunt, heavily colonised with coagulase-negative staphylococci. 2.5 ×

Subdivision within subgroup S.II was possible by a further biotyping procedure, many of the results of which were supported by Prof. Williams's phage typing. It was now revealed that

1. Two biotypes of S.II may co-exist in the blood and ventricular fluid.

2. The colonising biotype was usually present on the subject's skin and in nose and faeces.

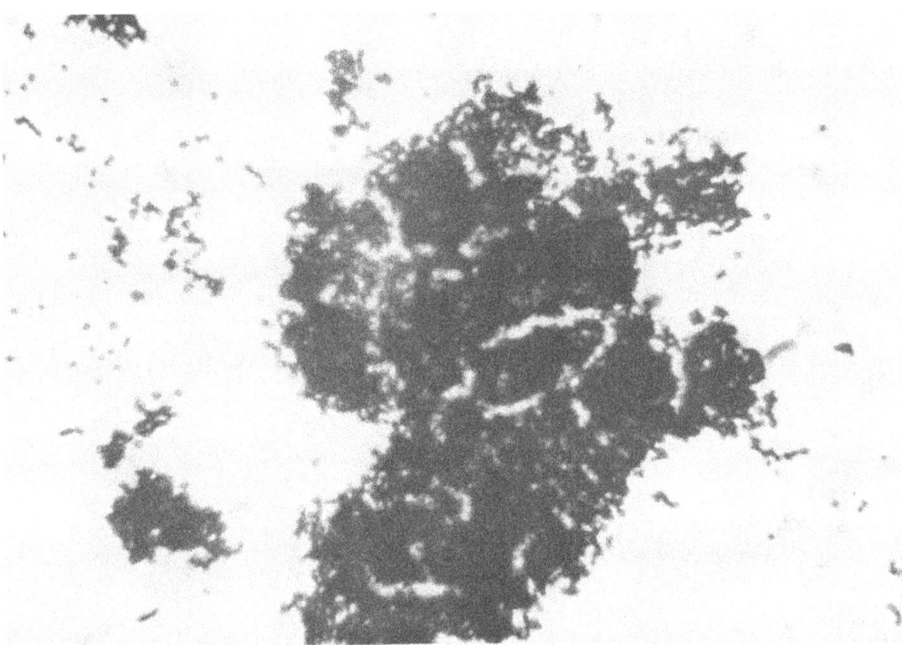

Fig. 3. *Gram film* of fluid from lightly colonised shunt lumen. 1,200 ×

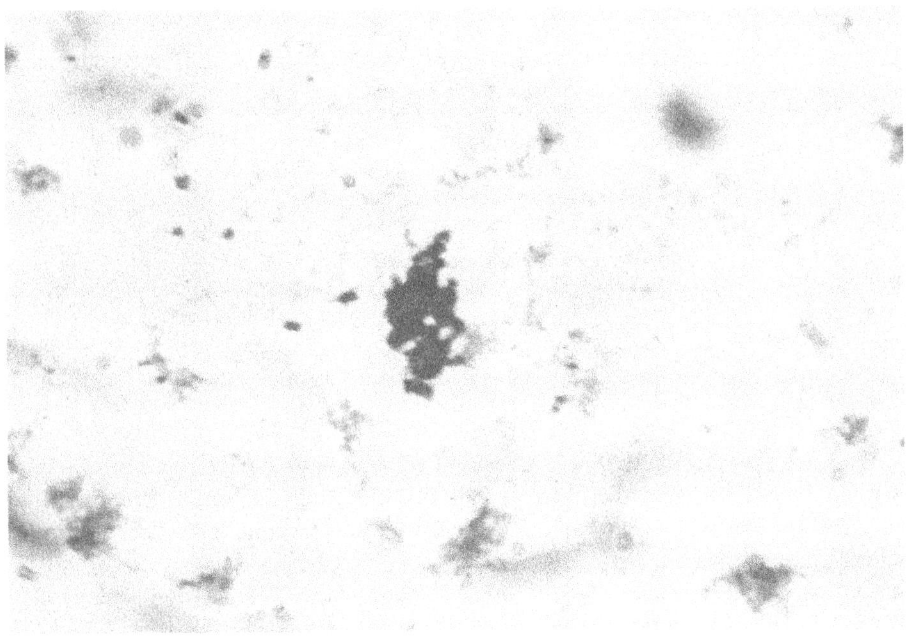

Fig. 4. *Gram film* of fluid from heavily colonised shunt lumen. 1,200 ×

3. After shunt replacement or manipulation, recolonisation was sometimes due to a different biotype.

These investigations left unanswered three major questions:

1. the routes of shunt colonisation,
2. the possibility of control or even prevention of colonisation, and
3. why S.II strains are so very prevalent in colonisation.

Table 1. *The classification of Micrococcaceae* (Baird-Parker, *1963*). *All are gram-positive, catalase-positive cocci*

Staphylococcus	S.I "*Staph. aureus*"
able to oxidise and ferment glucose	S.II
	S.III
	S.IV
	S.V
	S.VI
Micrococcus	M.1
able only to oxidise glucose	M.2
	M.3
	M.4
	M.5
	M.6
	M.7
	M.8

Sarcina unable to produce acid from glucose

Table 2. *The classification of Micrococcaceae from subjects in hospital*

Hospital patients and staff
701 strains of Micrococcaceae from 185 individuals
    84 % belonged to Staphylococcus genus
    50 % belonged to subgroup S.II

Babies in paedriatric surgical ward
$^{16}/_{17}$ babies had S.II on at least one body site

Staff in paediatric surgical ward
$^{9}/_{12}$ female staff had S.II on at least one body site

In brief, it seems likely that many shunt colonisations start with a bacteraemia, and the bacteria ascend the distal catheter to the shunt lumen, in time reaching the cerebral ventricles. The early recognition of bacteraemia is therefore of great clinical importance.

Nulsen and Becker (1966) observed that shunt colonisation was closely related to the positioning of the end of the distal catheter in the atrium and the risk of thrombus formation round the catheter following local trauma. The thrombi, even when very small, presumably attract transient bacteria and constitute a local reservoir. Results from the differential culture of the parts of excised colonised shunts tend to support the ascending theory. In the most recent 16 colonised shunts, 12 had staphylococci in all three sites, two had cocci in the distal catheter and lumen but not in the proximal catheter, and two had staphylococci in the distal catheter alone. The ascending theory is also supported by *in vitro* studies with a laboratory model of a shunt, when it was shown that S.II cocci

Table 3. *The classification of Micrococcaceae from persons not in hospital*

Infants, children and adults in normal domestic environs

326 strains from 50 individuals
67 % belonged to Staphylococcus genus
21 % belonged to subgroup S.II
$^6/_{10}$ babies (under 1 year) had S.II on at least one body site

Table 4. *Biotypes of Staphylococcus subgroup II from children with colonised valves*

Case No.	Biotypes recovered from						
	Blood	Shunt	Ventricular fluid	Axilla	Interscapular	Nose	Faeces
18	S.IIA	S.IIA	S.IIA	S.IIA[++]	S.IIA[++]	S.IIA[++]	S.IIA[+]
19	S.IIA	S.IIA	S.IIA	S.IIA[++]	S.V	S.V[+++]	S.IIA[+] S.V.[++]
20	S.IIA	S.IIA	S.IIA	S.IIA scanty	S.IIA scanty	S.IIA scanty M.2[++]	S.IIA[++]
21	S.IIA	S.IIA	S.IIA	S.IIA[++]	S.IIA[++]	S.IIA[+]	S.IIA scanty
	S.IIB	S.IIB		S.IIB[+]	S.IIB[+]	S.IIB[++]	
22	S.IIA	S.IIA S.IIG	Not examined	S.IIA[+] S.IIG[+]	No Staphs.	S.IIA[+++]	S.IIA scanty

could climb within 24 h from the bottom container to the shunt lumen, despite the downward flow of dilute nutrient broth, regulated to 1 ml/h through a low-pressure shunt; within 100 h the container simulating the ventricle was infected.

The treatment of established colonisation with antibiotics of the beta-lactam family has proved very unsuccessful, but it seems possible that perfusion of the shunt system with gentamicin, supported by adequate systemic dosage, may be more valuable. The very long-term prophylactic use of fucidin for the prevention of this complication is also contemplated.

The almost exclusive prevalence of subgroup S.II strains in shunt colonisation clearly merits thorough investigation. The production by staphylococci of two enzymes, *muramidase*, formerly called lysozyme, and *deoxyribonuclease* has been suggested by several workers as criteria of pathogenicity in addition to the traditional *coagulase* test, and shunt bacteria were accordingly tested.

The great majority of these colonising cocci possessed neither of the enzyme, and it may be that these organisms can stealthily and insidiously invade the prosthetic shunt from transient bacteraemias, without altering the somatic immune defences. Once established in the shunt, the colonisation constitutes a permanent

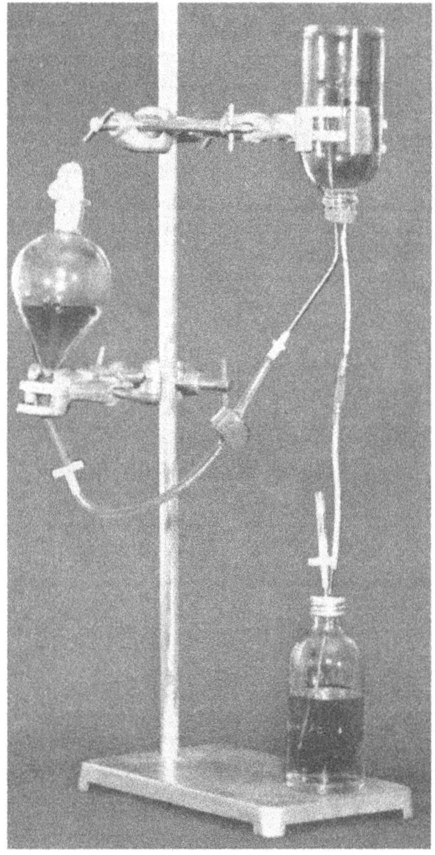

Fig. 5. Laboratory model of a ventriculo-atrial shunt. The lower container represented the heart atrium and the upper bottle the cerebral ventricle

reservoir for re-infection of the blood after the bacteraemia has been temporarily eliminated with antibacterial agents. Long experience has convinced us that the only sure therapy at present is the complete removal of the colonised shunt under heavy antibiotic cover, and its replacement at a later date.

The troublesome complication reported here involving an artificial internal prosthesis is, in a sense, an example of a man-made infection paralleled in nature by the colonisation with relatively harmless streptococci and staphylococci of damaged cardiac tissue. The greatly increasing use of many kinds of such prostheses makes it safe to predict that colonisation by relatively benign bacteria or by fungi will soon become a major laboratory and clinical problem.

Table 5. *Lysozyme production by staphylococci of clinical interest*

B-P subgroup	Origin	Total tested	Lysozyme production	
			positive	negative
S.I	Septic skin lesions	100	100	0
S.II	Colonised V-A shunts	40	3 (weak)	37
S.II	Wounds	3	0	3
S.II	Prosthetic heart valves	6	0	6
S.III	Prosthetic heart valves	2	0	2

Table 6. *DN.ase production by staphylococci of clinical interest*

B-P subgroup	Orogon	Total tested	DN.ase production	
			positive	negative
S.II	Septic skin lesions	50	50	0
S.II	Colonised V-A shunts	26	0	26
S.II	Wounds	1	1	2
S.II	Prosthetic heart valves	6	1	5
S.III	Prosthetic heart valves	2	0	2

References

BAIRD-PARKER, A. C.: A classification of micrococci and staphylococci based on physiological and biochemical tests. J. gen. Microbiol. 38, 363 (1963).
NULSEN, F. E., BECKER, D. P.: Workshop in hydrocephalus. Proceedings 1965 (SHULMAN, K., Ed.), Univ. of Pennsylvania, School of Medicine, Philadelphia.

Dr. R. J. HOLT
Queen Mary's Hospital for Children
Group Laboratories
Carshalton, Surrey, England

Discussion

KASS: An analogy to the data on tooth extraction is warranted. The issue of prophylaxis here is so terribly crucial, so one might review some of the data on prophylaxis in relation to tooth extractions and raise some questions in relation to the problem. First, are SII strains the major staphylococcal flora of the gingiva? Second, what is found in the blood of individuals after they chew vigorously for a few minutes (which is a classical way of getting the dental flora to show up in the blood)? In small babies, such as those Dr. HOLT studies, can one detect bacteremia soon after they have been fed? Third, and perhaps most important, one should call attention to what happened in the prophylaxis of tooth extractions. Where alpha streptococci were dominant in the blood after extraction of a tooth without prophylaxis, the use of either penicillin or tetracycline reduced the number of bacteremias substantially, but the organisms that were found in the blood after prophylaxis were staphylococci and enterococci. This is poor comfort to those who would like to use prophylaxis to reduce the rate of endocarditis.

HOLT: This will come up in debate tomorrow, I am sure. But, to set the scene once more, we have got to define the kind of prophylaxis. I imagine that dental prophylaxis may be short-term; I am thinking here of the very long-term prophylaxis with low but adequate dosage. We have already had a lot of experience of this with cystic fibrosis; very much in trepidation, Dr. DAVID LAWSON, who is the director of our Cystic Fibrosis Research Unit, in 1964 started to put all of his cases on cloxacillin for ever onwards and everybody thought this was very heroic and possibly dangerous. He was utterly convinced, and we were convinced as well, that it is *Staphyloccus aureus* which is the root of most of the chest trouble with cystic fibrosis and that the gram-negatives, and occasionally *Candida*, are superimposed on this. We then felt he was right, and clinically, we believe now he is right, because we are now seeing much healthier 6-year old and 7-year old cystic fibrosis children than we have ever seen before. However, there may be other factors here. Neither have we seen the severity of chest infection when it did occur. We have searched repeatedly for cloxacillin-resistant staphylococci in these cases and have not found them. This perhaps is considered heresy.

KASS: It is not the worst of heresies. The way to find out in cystic fibrosis, whether cloxacillin or anything else works, is a properly controlled trial. I believe that the data, as presently available, cannot be completely evaluated because the methods for detecting cystic fibrosis have become so much more sensitive in recent years, so that we are treating a much healthier group of children. It is no surprise, therefore, that children nowadays are doing better. That is why the properly controlled trial is essential.

HOLT: I think we were among the pioneers in the very early detection of cystic fibrosis and I think, therefore, that LAWSON's experience, clinical and bacteriological, is valid. He, of course, was aware as we were also, that there *should* be a controlled trial, but it is the old problem of who is going to decide which is which; who is going to withhold literally life-saving procedures if you believe strongly enough in them!

KASS: If one believes completely that the treatment is life-saving, then one should not be the one to do a controlled trial. Those who think it is not life-saving, or have some doubts, are the ones who should conduct the trial.

HOLT: Yes, that is a valid point.

NAUMANN: I have to confirm your poor results in the treatment of colonisation from our own material with the penicillins, including intraventricular application.

Therefore, I am extremely surprised at the good effects you report with gentamicin. Would you give us more detailed information on your gentamicin therapy, especially on the dosage and route of application!

HOLT: The lumen of the shunt was exteriorised—the central part just under the skin. This was the Azygos shunt which, as I explained, we had to do something about or lose out completely. Then, as far as I remember, 20 mg of gentamicin were run into the lumen.

NAUMANN: Per day?

HOLT: No, just in one dose very slowly, with a very fine hair-like needle, because we dare not damage the plastic wall of the lumen. We had to make sure that it did not leak, otherwise we risk a horrible "tract infection" as well. This was very slowly perfused down 24 h before we started a relatively heavy systemic course of gentamicin, with something like 3 mg/kg/day. We maintained that course for a further week and in this particular case it succeeded. I assayed serum about 2 h after the massive dose; of course we got very high levels of gentamicin quite out of proportion to the systemic levels that are expected during normal gentamicin therapy.

ERICSSON: Have you checked thoroughly the toxicity of gentamicin as to the hearing of these infants.

HOLT: Yes. We started gentamicin in 1967 and we were aware of this risk and, as far as it is possible to test the ototoxicity effect on small children, our people are quite sure that there has been *no* damage. We think it is only the prolonged therapy that causes this. Perhaps Prof. MARGET could give us some ideas on this, as I can see that you think it is ototoxic.

FINLAND: I wonder if Dr. HOLT or Prof. WILLIAMS have data on *Staphylococcus albus (Staph. epidermidis)* obtained from bacterial endocarditis, which is a common disease, particularly in addicts, and perhaps represents about half of all cases, especially of staphylococcal endocarditis. Dr. HOLT, do you have any data?

HOLT: I would really like to have some staphylococci from these cases and if anybody has got any we would like to type them.

FINLAND: Prof. WILLIAMS, do you have any information about this?

WILLIAMS: I do not think we have any strains from addicts; we have a few staphylococci from post-operative endocarditis and all of these have been of the serotype SII.

PULVERER: We are working now in this field and hope to have good results next year.

FINLAND: I hope that we can obtain some of the material for the bio-classification because, as I indicated, we became interested in *Staph. epidermidis* when Dr. KJELLANDER was in our laboratory, and Dr. SABATH is now continuing that interest. At the moment we have not seen an increase in incidence of resistant strains of *Staph. epidermidis*, but that was the first place where we found methicillin-resistance. I am not sure about cloxacillin-resistance, except that all our strains that are methicillin-resistant also have decreased sensitivity to cloxacillin. Some years ago, Dr. McCARTHY in my laboratory started to develop a phage system for *Staphylococcus epidermidis* and we studied about a thousand strains and developed half a dozen phages, but unfortunately, he left and I have never got up the courage to start this up again. I am glad BLAIRD-PARKER and WILLIAMS have and I hope to take advantage of their experience.

DASCHNER: As far as ototoxicity of gentamicin in the treatment of cystic fibrosis is concerned, Dr. L. L. CAUSAY presented a paper at the last Interscience Conference in Chicago, describing about 60 patients treated with a course of about 12 g of intermittent therapy. She never found any ototoxicity.

CHABBERT: I should answer your question about resistance of *Staph. epidermidis* to methicillin because we have a lot of that in Paris. Surprisingly about one-third of them are not penicillinase producers; they are only methicillin-resistant without penicillinase.

HOLT: I published a similar observation in about 1966, that a number of coagulase negative staphylococci were resistant to penicillin and to cloxacillin and yet did not produce penicillinase. This seemed to us an example of the "intrinsic" resistance that we always suspected but have never been able to find in *Staph. aureus*.

Bayer-Symposium III, 91—96 (1971)

Pathogenic Significance
of Coagulase-Negative Staphylococci

G. PULVERER and J. PILLICH

With 2 Figures

Coagulase-activity is today accepted as the best in vitro-test for proof of staphylococcal pathogenicity. Coagulase-positive staphylococci are considered to be pathogens, coagulase-negative staphylococci as non-pathogens.

Synonyms are: *S. aureus* or *S. pyogenes* for coagulase-positive staphylococci, *S. albus* or *S. epidermidis* or *S. saprophyticus* for coagulase-negative staphylococci.

This differentiation is, of course, very useful for diagnosis in routine work. But there is an important disadvantage: coagulase-negative staphylococci, considered as non-pathogens, are often regarded as secondary contaminants, when cultivated from infections. This is not always correct, because today there is no doubt that coagulase-negative staphylococci can also cause infections.

Coagulase-negative staphylococci have been found as pathogens in different infections. In 1967 we collected and discussed all reports related to this (PULVERER and HALSWICK).

We found 128 cases of endocarditis due to *S. albus*, mostly after heart surgery, but certainly the real number of cases must be much higher. BRANDT and SWAHN for example, calculated that *S. albus* might now be responsible for more than 1% of all cases of endocarditis.

After neurosurgery, especially in connexion with hydrocephalus, coagulase-negative staphylococci are not infrequently proved to be the cause of complications. The same applies to wound infections: WILSON and STUART reported that *S. albus* was found in pure culture in 53 out of 1,200 cases of wound infections (4.4%).

Coagulase-negative staphylococci are most frequently cultivated in cases of urinary tract infections. PEREIRA calculated that 9% of all urinary tract infections in Portugal are caused by staphylococci, in 43% of these cases by *S. albus*.

ROBERTS examined samples of urine collected by suprapubic punction and he could demonstrate S. albus in six cases of urinary tract infections. In 1969 MABECK proved *S. albus* to be the causative agent in 31 of 219 women with bacteriuria.

MORTENSEN stated that a negative coagulase-reaction of a staphylococcus does not exclude this strain as a cause of urinary tract infection.

What is the *S. albus*-situation in the Cologne region?

Table 1 shows how often we cultivated coagulase-negative staphylococci from samples of pyogenic infections. In 1960 *S. albus* was present in 8.6% of all samples; in the first 6 months of 1970 it got up to 13.5%. It is very remarkable that *S. albus* was found in pure culture in more than half of the samples.

The occurrence of *S. albus* in samples from urinary tract infections is presented in Table 2. As compared with 1960, coagulase-negative staphylococci decreased from 5.4 to 3.4% in 1969; almost half of the samples showed *S. albus* in pure culture.

There is no doubt that coagulase-negative staphylococci have pathogenic potentialities in some cases. However, there is also no doubt that *S. albus* must be considered as a contaminant in other cases. So the cultivation of *S. albus* raises the dilemma what to do with this diagnosis. Therefore, it would be very important

Table 1. *Coagulase-negative staphylococci in pyogenic infections*

Year	Samples examined	Coagulase-negative staphylococci	Of these in pure culture %
1960	2,266	196 = 8.6 %	53
1969 January—June	2,129	220 = 10.3 %	58
1969 July—December	2,330	297 = 12.8 %	65
1970 January—June	2,114	286 = 13.5 %	57

Table 2. *Coagulase-negative staphylococci in urinary tract infections*

Year	Samples examined	Coagulase-negative staphylococci	Of these in pure culture %
1960	1,511	82 = 5.4 %	51
1969	14,569	497 = 3.4 %	46

to find some reliable markers with which we can differentiate between facultative pathogenic strains of *S. albus* and really non-pathogenic coagulase-negative staphylococci.

In 1962 Reitler and Seligman investigated the precipitating property of staphylococci on plasma agar. Coagulase-negative staphylococci from infections showed a positive reaction more often (67.2%) than strains from normal material (28.6%). Jacobs, Willis and Goodburn in 1964 found that 5 of 227 coagulase-negative staphylococci produced detectable amounts of deoxyribonuclease. They believed that these strains may be representatives of the coagulase-negative organisms that are occasionally found to cause infections in man.

In 1965 Ivler compared coagulase-negative strains from endocarditis and from the nose. He found that coagulase-negative staphylococci associated with cases of endocarditis had endogenous respiration values comparable to those of

S. aureus. In the same year Quinn, Cox and Fisher investigated three groups of strains of *S. albus:*

1. Strains from cases with bacteremia.

2. Strains found in pure culture of open wound infections.

3. Strains from nasal cultures.

They took into consideration the following tests: colony-morphology, coagulase and catalase activities, fermentation of glucose and mannitol, penicillinase activity and pathogenicity for mice. The three groups of coagulase-negative staphylococci showed no differences.

In 1968 Kleck and Donahue examined 106 strains of *S. albus* from nasal carriers and 35 from clinical material; 22 of these 35 strains were from cases of endocarditis. They concluded: coagulase-negative cultures obtained from the normal nasal flora of humans and from clinical sources are similar in their biochemical characteristics and in their ability to produce hemolysins.

Likewise, Mitchell failed to demonstrate any correlation between Baird-Parker's subgroups and participation in infections. Also in 1968, Spink and Strong tried to differentiate between really apathogenic and potentially pathogenic strains of *S. albus*. The following tests were of no help: hemolysin- and phosphatase-activities, resistance to polymyxin and to human serum, cultivation at 43°, and enrichment in NaCl-broth. However, egg-yolk-activity and fermentation of mannitol showed some differences: half the strains from clinical material were mannitol-positive and egg-yolk-negative. On the other hand, half the strains from ears, nostrils, and eyes were mannitol-negative and egg-yolk-positive.

In 1969, Mortensen divided 46 coagulase-negative strains from urinary tract infections into two groups, according to fermentation of glucose. In the same year, Smith and Farkas-Himsley compared the following strains: 21 coagulase-negative staphylococci from infections (20 cases of endocarditis, 1 case of post-operative meningitis), 5 strains of *S. aureus*, 2 coagulase-negative variants of *S. aureus* and 5 coagulase-negative nonpathogenic staphylococci. They analysed the findings with respect to 46 factors. The coagulase-negative strains from infections constituted a group that fitted between *S. aureus* and the non-pathogenic *S. albus*. The authors concluded: if a species must be designated under the present system of classification, a strain producing coagulase can be called *S. aureus*. However, strains lacking this character cannot be classified with accuracy as *S. epidermidis*.

Half a year ago we started a similar study. Our investigations are not yet finished, so we can give only a preliminary report. We investigated three groups of staphylococci:

1. 100 strains of *S. aureus* from clinical sources.

2. 50 strains of *S. epidermidis* from human nasal carriers.

3. 101 coagulase-negative staphylococci isolated from infections; 46 strains of the last group were received gratefully from Mortensen in Denmark, 20 additional strains from Smith and Farkas-Himsley in Canada, 35 strains were isolated in our laboratory: 18 from cases of urinary tract infections and 17 from pyogenic infections, such as, osteomylitis, bacteremia, furunculosis, adnexitis and hydro-

cephalus subjected to surgery. All three groups of staphylococci were classified according to recommendations of the International Sub-committee of Taxonomy.

Coagulase-activity was tested with rabbit plasma, also according to the above recommendations. Phage typing was performed with the International set of *Staphylococcus aureus* phages, using phages in $1{,}000 \times$ RTD. Lysogeny of all strains was proved on six indicator-strains. As stated in a previous publication (PULVERER, SCZUKA and PILLICH) these indicator-strains 57, 879, 67 K, 54 K, C 17 and C 938 are strains of *S. aureus* of human origin.

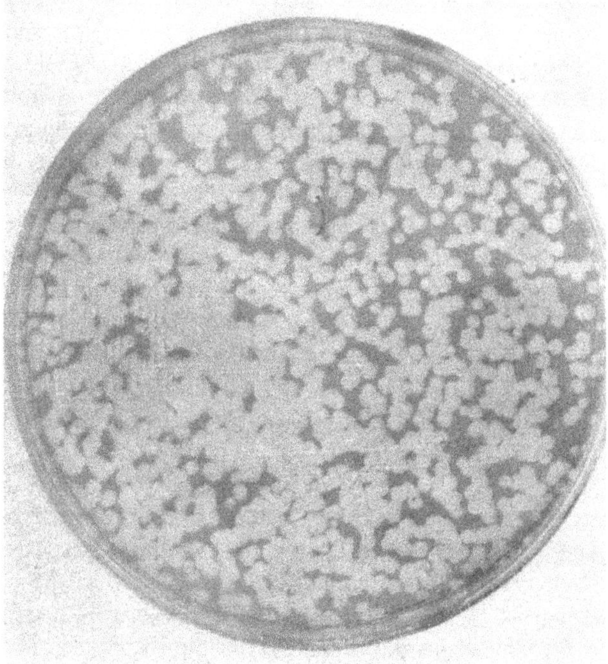

Fig. 1. Typical phage-reaction with polyvalent phages

Sensitivity of all strains to polyvalent phages was examined, using the phages 131, A5 and A3 in RTD. Here three types of reactions were possible:

1. No reaction with any of the three phages.

2. At least one of the three phages 131, A5 and A3 gave a typical phage-reaction (see Fig. 1).

3. At least one of the three phages produced atypical phage plaques (see Fig. 2).

Table 3 shows our preliminary results. There are two remarkable points:

1. 10% of the coagulase-negative strains from Denmark could be typed with the International set of phages in $1{,}000 \times$ RTD.

2. The three polyvalent phages 131, A5 and A3 reacted with all the strains of *S. aureus* in RTD but with no strain of the non-pathogenic *S. epidermidis*-group.

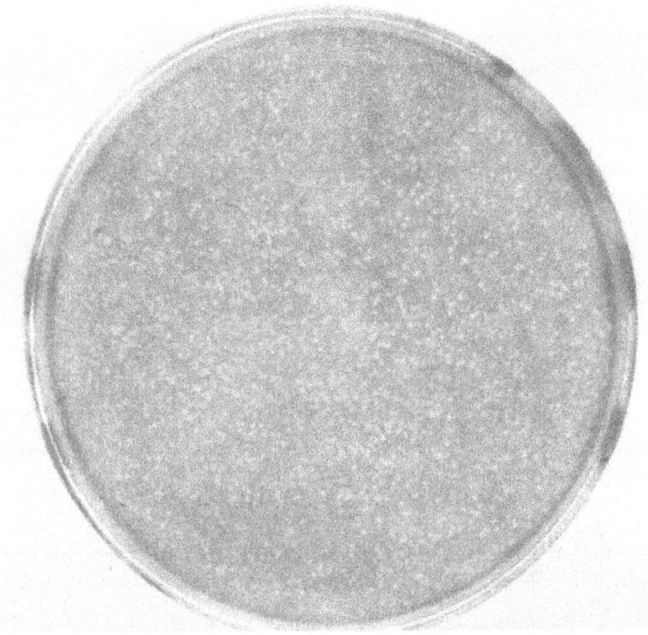

Fig. 2. Atypical phage-reaction with polyvalent phages

Table 3. *Relation of pathogenic coagulase-negative staphylococci to S. aureus and S. epidermidis*

	Number of strains	Coagulase	Phage typing %	Lysogeny %	Sensitivity to polyvalent phages	
					typical reaction %	atypical reaction %
S. aureus	100	+	75	100	100	–
S. epidermidis	50	–	–	–	–	–
Pathogenic coagulase-negative staphylococci						
Denmark	46	–	10	–	7	–
Canada	20	–	–	–	20	10
Germany	35	–	–	–	20	15

+ = positive, – = negative.

On the other hand, at least some of the coagulase-negative staphylococci from clinical material showed reactions. Counting typical and atypical reaction together, the sensitivity of the polyvalent phages ranged between 7 % of the Danish strains to 35 % of the Cologne strains.

As already mentioned, our studies are not yet finished. We also started investigations on lysogeny, using coagulase-negative indicator-strains, and on phage-typing with phages isolated from strains of *S. albus*. We are also doing genetic studies, subgrouping according to Baird-Parker; we are establishing the DNA-composition and trying to perform statistical analyses. We hope to have clear and exact results next year.

At the moment we can give the following conclusions: Coagulase-negative staphylococci do not represent a homogenous group with respect to the pathogenic capacity of strains.

It looks as if the facultatively pathogenic strains of *S. albus* constitute an intermediary group between *S. aureus* and the really non-pathogenic strains of *S. albus*. Furthermore, it seems to be possible to find in vitro tests for differentiating these two groups of *S. albus*.

References

Brandt, L., Swahn, B.: Subacute bacterial endocarditis due to coagulase-negative *Staphylococcus albus*. Acta med. scand. **166**, 125—132 (1960).

Ivler, D.: Comparative metabolism of virulent and avirulent staphylococci. Ann. N.Y. Acad. Sci. **128**, 62—79 (1965).

Jacobs, S. I., Willis, A. T., Goodburn, G. M.: Pigment production and enzymatic activity of staphylococci: the differentiation of pathogens from commensals. J. Path. Bact. **87**, 151—156 (1964).

Kleck, J. L., Donahue, J. A.: Production of thermostable hemolysin by cultures of *Staphylococcus epidermidis*. J. infect. Dis. **118**, 317—323 (1968).

Mabeck, C. E.: Significance of coagulase-negative staphylococcal bacteriuria. Lancet **1969 II**, 1150—1152.

Mitchell, R. G.: Classification of *Staphylococcus albus* strains isolated from the urinary tract. J. clin. Path. **21**, 93—96 (1968).

Mortensen, N.: Studies in urinary tract infections. III. Biochemical characteristics of coagulase-negative staphylococci associated with urinary tract infections. Acta med. scand. **186**, 47—51 (1969).

Pereira, A. T.: Coagulase-negative strains of Staphylococcus possessing antigen 51 as agents of urinary tract infections. J. clin. Path. **15**, 252—253 (1962).

Pulverer, G., Halswick, R.: Coagulase-negative Staphylokokken *(Staphylococcus albus)* als Krankheitserreger. Dtsch. med. Wschr. **92**, 1141—1145 (1967).

— Sczuka, Ch., Pillich, J.: Lysogenitätsuntersuchungen an pathogenen Staphylokokken von Mensch und Tier. I. Differenzierung mit Hilfe von 6 Indikatorstämmen menschlicher Herkunft. Zbl. Bakt. I. Abt. Orig. **203**, 277—291 (1967).

Quinn, E. L., Cox, F., Fisher, M.: The problem of associating coagulase-negative staphylococci with disease. Ann. N.Y. Acad. Sci. **128**, 428—442 (1965).

Reitler, R., Seligman, R.: Precipitation in plasma-agar and pathogenicity of coagulase-negative *Staphylococcus albus*. Israel med. J. **21**, 225—228 (1962).

Roberts, A. P.: Micrococcaceae from the urinary tract in pregnancy. J. clin. Path. **20**, 631—632 (1967).

Smith, H. B. H., Farkas-Himsley, H.: The relationship of pathogenic coagulase-negative staphylococci to *Staphylococcus aureus*. Canad. J. Microbiol. **15**, 879—890 (1969).

Spink, M. S., Strong, Sh.: The pathogenic variety of *Staphylococcus albus*. J. path. Bact. **95**, 295—299 (1968).

Wilson, T. S., Stuart, R. D.: *Staphylococcus albus* in wound infection and in septicemia. Canad. med. Ass. J. **93**, 8—16 (1965).

Prof. Dr. G. Pulverer
Direktor des Hygiene-Instituts
der Universität Köln
D-5000 Köln-Lindenthal
Fürst-Pückler-Straße 56

Discussion

HOLT: I think it is important to differentiate between the staphylococci which are proven to have caused urinary tract infection and those which colonize prostheses, and here the lysozyme muramidase test and the deoxyribonuclease test may be of use. I collected 37 urinary coagulase-negative strains from MORTENSEN, from MITCHELL and from ROBERTS and, on lysozyme testing, 20 of the 37 were positive. It is interesting that MITCHELL and MORTENSEN both found that the Micrococcus 3 (M3) strains were very common in proven urinary tract infection and of those 13 M's recovered from the urinary tract, 11 were lysozyme positive. When we examined random M3's from skin and from nose, mainly from skin of healthy people, then perhaps one-third of 15 strains were positive. Of the DNA's activity, again the 37 coagulase-negative staphylococci were examined, and 10 were DNA-positive, which is a far higher percentage than one would normally expect. I exclude *Staphylococcus aureus* from this series; these were all S2 to S6 in the BAIRD-PARKER scheme and then M1 to M8.

PULVERER: We are testing all these factors, all factors that you can imagine, for numerical analysis, but at the moment I cannot say whether they are really good factors or not. We are also testing for lysostaphin-sensitivity and for all other factors; we have collected them and have put them into a computer program.

KASS: Are there any data about urethral staphylococci? I am not sure that the organisms from the skin are the ones to look at when considering urinary tract strains.

PULVERER: At the moment I cannot say.

HOLT: Very little indeed, mine is entirely a children's hospital and this problem does not normally arise. We have only had about three cases of this type of infection so that I am entirely dependent upon people from adult hospitals to supply them and clearly one has to take their word. As to the urethral and perineal staphylococci, I have done very little work on them. The skin strains were obtained from swabbings of the interscapular region.

KASS: Unfortunately, the majority of strains that are ascribed to the urinary tract as pathogens turn out not to have caused anything. One might ask whether the strains colonizing the urethra and the ones which ultimately affect the urinary tract are in any way different, or whether they are the same organisms as those found elsewhere in the same individual.

Bayer-Symposium III, 99—109 (1971)
© by Springer-Verlag 1971

Changes in the Virulence and Antibiotic Resistance of *Staphylococcus aureus*

R. E. O. WILLIAMS

With 5 Figures

Evidence for Changes in Virulence

The establishment of long-term changes in the virulence of any pathogenic microbe is difficult and, for *Staphylococcus aureus* the difficulties are enhanced by the fact that there is so little quantitative evidence on the incidence of staphylococcal disease, which is, for the most part, neither lethal nor statutorily reportable.

Of the diseases that are recorded in the national mortality statistics two, namely "osteomyelitis" and "carbuncles and boils", may probably be regarded as virtually exclusively due to staphylococcal infection. The numbers of deaths recorded under these two headings in England and Wales for 1920 to 1968 are shown in Fig. 1. The most striking feature is, naturally, the dramatic fall in mortality during the 1940's, doubtless attributable to the introduction of penicillin, which became reasonably well available in Britain from about 1945. The apparent increase in mortality for both causes between 1920 and 1935 is curious and does not, so far as I know, have any obvious explanation. Nor is it clear whether the fall between 1935 and 1945 could be attributable to the use of the early sulphonamides (the dramatic effect of which on puerperal sepsis is illustrated for comparison in Fig. 1) or whether it represents a spontaneous reversal of the trend of the period 1920 to 1935.

Figures presented by RAVENHOLT (1962) for mortality from suppurative disease in Seattle, U.S.A. between 1905 and 1960 showed a general fall in mortality over the whole period, with some indication of an increased rate of fall between 1940 and 1950; his figures, however, certainly included some non-staphylococcal disease.

In Norway, national statistics on the incidence of pemphigus neonatorum, quoted by LINDAU and LÖFKVIST (1958), showed a dramatic rise during the 1940's.

During the last 30 years interest in staphylococcal infection has been centred mainly on post-operative infection of surgical wounds and infections of mothers and infants in maternity hospitals, but it is unfortunately very difficult to extract from the published records any long-term indications of changes in the behaviour of staphylococci, independent of changes in the management of patients. One or two studies of the incidence of infection in comparable series of surgical wounds have indicated remarkably little secular change; for example, BARNES et al. (1959, 1962) analysed infections after appendectomy, herniorrhaphy and hysterectomy over a 20-year period and found no real trends. On the other hand HOWE (1956) recorded a progressive increase in one hospital between 1949 and 1953, followed by a decline in incidence. LIDWELL and his colleagues (1970) have documented a rise in the incidence of staphylococcal wound sepsis in patients nursed in one surgical ward over the period 1956 to 1967. This rise was associated with the spread in the ward during the latter part of the period of staphylococci with the phage pattern 84/85.

Some published figures that we (WILLIAMS et al., 1966, p. 80) collected show very substantial variations in post-operative infection rates from different units, but no evidence of a systematic change with time.

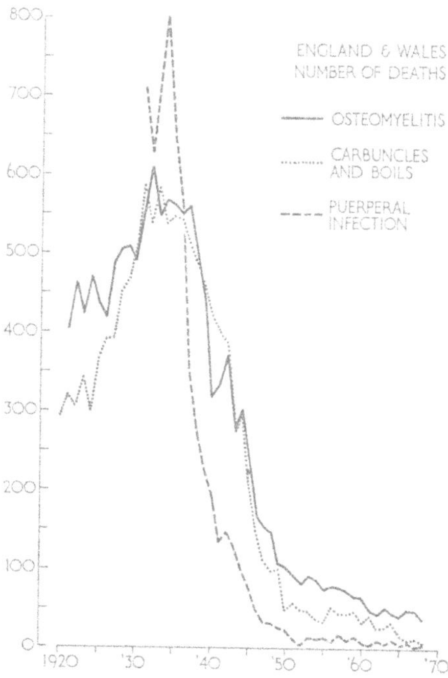

Fig. 1. Numbers of deaths attributed to osteomyelitis (————), carbuncle (......) and puerperal infection (- - - - -), England and Wales 1921—1968 (from Annual Reports of Registrar General)

Clearly the data on the incidence of staphylococcal disease give only a very inadequate picture, but there seems no evidence for massive changes in infections in the community generally, such as have been seen with enteric fever, or scarlet fever. Hospital records are even more difficult to interpret than national mortality records, but there appears to be no real evidence for great changes in staphylococcal disease.

And yet a glance at the indices of the world's medical journals of the 1950's would suggest that we were being struck by a severe pandemic of staphylococcal infection. Was this simply new recognition of a long-standing situation? Or, if there were changes in the disease not recognizable from the statistics, was it a decline in the hygienic precautions in hospitals (brought about, as the virtuous always claimed, by the "abuse" of antibiotics)? Or was it a change in the staphylococci that happened to be prevalent? I believe that all three factors contributed to the picture of the 1950's, but in this communication emphasis must be given to the last. Pointers are given by examination of the records of phage typing.

Phage Types of Staphylococcus aureus

Phage typing of staphylococci was generally employed from the early 1950's and it soon became clear that there were ecological differences between the three principal broad phage "groups" (WILLIAMS, RIPPON and DOWSETT, 1953). With more experience it became clear that at least in one hospital, staphylococci of different phage types varied very substantially in their pathogenic ability. A few appeared to be able to spread among the patients and to cause disease; others were able to spread and colonize patients but rarely caused any disease; some that could certainly cause disease in individuals rarely spread to other patients; and many were introduced into the ward by carriers but neither spread nor caused disease (SHOOTER et al., 1958). Analysis of the material sent to the Staphylococcal Reference Laboratory confirmed these conclusions and demonstrated that, in the years 1954 to 1957, staphylococci with no more than six phage patterns accounted for over half the "epidemics" of staphylococcal infection recognized in hospitals in Britain (WILLIAMS, 1959). Dominant among these "epidemic types" was, of course, "type 80/81" (see also FEKETY and BENNETT, 1959).

Change in Phage-Type Distribution

The distribution over the main groups recognized by phage typing of staphylococci isolated from hospital patients in several surveys is shown in Fig. 2. Around 1950, 40 to 50% of the strains fell into group III, in which were found most of the early antibiotic-resistant staphylococci, and 10 to 15% were in group I. Five years later, both in Britain and the United States, the situation had changed profoundly, thanks to the appearance of type 80/81. By 1966, the situation had altered again, with the virtual disappearance of type 80/81.

The changes are seen more dramatically in the surveys carried out by the Public Health Laboratory Service, Staphylococcus Reference Laboratory, at Colindale, London (Fig. 3). Until 1959 the figures are based on staphylococci sent to the laboratory from incidents thought to represent hospital-acquired infection(JEVONS and PARKER, 1964); after 1960 they are derived from a survey of staphylococci from a random selection of infected lesions in eight London hospitals (HEWITT, BROCK and PARKER, personal communication, 1970). During the 15 years covered by these surveys the dominant staphylococci have changed several times. Strains with the phage pattern 80 (later 80/81), which were first described by ROUNTREE and FREEMAN (1955) in Australia, were recognized in Britain in 1954 and rapidly became the outstanding hospital staphylococci, reaching a peak of prevalence in 1958. From 1957 onwards there was a great increase in the prevalence of strains typing as 52/52A/80/81 and subsequently a decline in 80/81. These strains were succeeded in Britain and several European countries (but not in the United States)

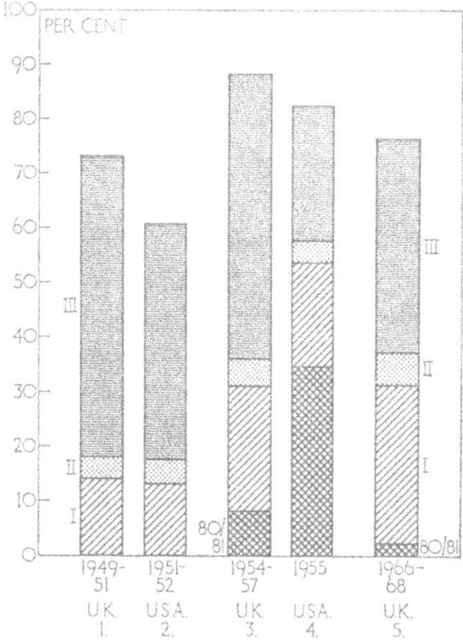

Fig. 2. Phage types of staphylococci from hospital patients: *1* WILLIAMS, RIPPON and DOW-
SETT (1953); *2* and *4* WALLMARK and FINLAND (1961); *3* WILLIAMS (1959); *5* HEWITT, BROCK
and PARKER (pers. communication, 1970)

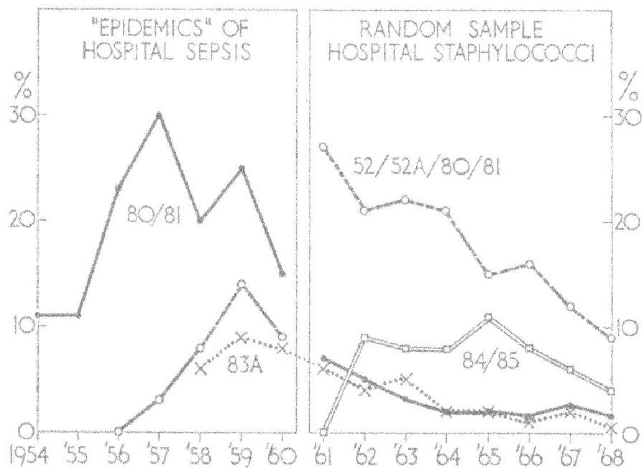

Fig. 3. Changes in prevalence of some phage types of staphylococci. Figures for 1954—1960
from JEVONS and PARKER (1964). Figures for 1961—1968 by HEWITT, BROCK and PARKER
(pers. communication, 1970)

by strains lysed by phage 83A; and later these in turn gave way to a complex
group of strains, many of which are typically lysed by two new phages 84 and 85.

The succession of types is also particularly well illustrated on strains from
patients with bacteraemia in Denmark. Fig. 4 is based on the Danish material

published by JESSEN et al. (1969) and supplemented by a personal communication from Dr. K. ROSENDAL (1970). A striking feature of the succession of phage types has been a substantial degree of synchrony in various parts of the world. The strains typing as 80/81 were recognized as a major epidemic variety in Australia, the United States and Canada, Britain, Denmark and many other European countries during the years 1954 to 1958, and where phage typing had been practised for long enough, it was clear that there had been a real increase in the prevalence of the strains during the previous few years.

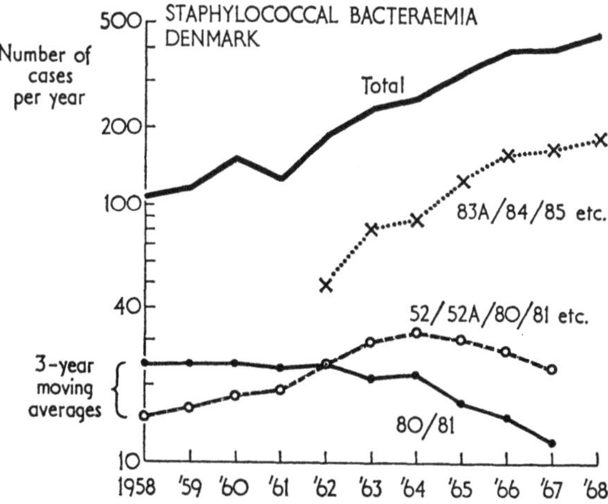

Fig. 4. Changes in phage types of staphylococci from patients with bacteraemia (JESSEN et al., 1969 and pers. communication from Dr. K. ROSENDAL, 1970)

Clearly there have been changes in the dominant staphylococci over the last two decades. One may consider first the mechanism of the change; second, the possible reasons for it, and third any possible consequences.

Mechanism of Change in Phage Type

To some extent, the changes in the phage patterns seen in staphylococci result from a change in the staphylococci, namely lysogenization by a type-determining phage. That this was a possible explanation for the change from the pattern 80/81 to 52/52A/80/81 was shown by ASHESHOV and RIPPON (1959) and by ROUNTREE (1959). Convincing evidence that the same phenomenon was concerned in the production of strains of the 84/85 complex from strains typing as 83A was offered by JEVONS, JOHN and PARKER (1966), who also showed clearly that the change must have taken place on many occasions and effected the conversion of a whole series of slightly differing strains typing as 83A.

BÜLOW (1968) documented a similar phenomenon in the staphylococci from a hospital in Denmark. Staphylococci typable only with a new phage, "6557" (which is certainly closely related to phages 84 and 85), were apparently derived from strains previously typed as 83A, or with some other group III pattern, by lysogenization with a blocking phage. He has subsequently produced evidence (BÜLOW, 1970) for the "epidemic spread" of the blocking phages among the 83A strains and related phage-group III strains in hospitals and has suggested that this process was responsible not only for the change in phage type but also for the change to neomycin- and bacitracin-resistance.

BÜLOW refers to epidemic spread of phages but does not discuss the mechanism by which such spread could occur. No one has produced evidence for the dispersal of free phage by carriers of lysogenic staphylococci, and such a phenomenon seems inherently improbable. It is more likely that the phage exchange occurs when two different strains of staphylococci together colonize a carrier site or wound, but there is clearly a need for some more direct evidence on this process.

It is reasonable to conclude that some of the changes in the dominant phage patterns represent typing changes in the prevalent staphylococci rather than replacement of one strain by another. This cannot, however, explain all the changes observed: it is highly unlikely that a strain typing as 52/52A/80/81 could be converted to one typing as 83A; the latter might, however, have arisen from some other strain of group III, of which there have always been a great variety in circulation in hospitals.

Whether 80/81 arose once and spread over practically the whole world, or whether strains with the same characteristics arose in several places, will never be known for certain, though ASHESHOV and WINKLER (1966) consider that, because all strains typing as 80/81 are lysogenic both for a group F phage and also for a completely defective phage that blocks the reaction with phages 52 and 52A, all must have had a common origin. BLAIR and CARR (1960) reported that they had found many strains typing as 80/81 in a collection of staphylococci isolated before 1947, but it appears from their paper that virtually all the strains included under the heading 80/81 were in fact lysed by phages 52 or 52A, or both, as well, and in this way differed from the "true 80/81".

There can be little doubt that the change from 80/81 to 52/52A/80/81 has occurred on many occasions as has the conversion of 83A strains to one or other of the 84/85 complex.

Causes of the Change in Phage Type Distributions

The changes in the relative prevalence of the different phage types might be due to variations in the inherent communicability and virulence of the staphylococci, or they might be due to selection by the antibiotics used in hospitals. There can be little doubt that both factors have played a part.

It seems very likely that the high frequency of phage-group III strains in hospitals around 1950 (Fig. 2) was due, in part, to the fact that, at that time, most antibiotic-resistant strains fell into that phage group. On a limited scale neomycin prophylaxis was found to alter the distribution of staphylococci in a burns unit (LOWBURY et al., 1964), and it seems very likely that the neomycin-resistance of the "84/85" strains was an important feature in favouring their spread, which occurred at a time when neomycin nasal creams and sprays were being widely used (ALDER and GILLESPIE, 1967).

But it does not seem that differences in antibiotic sensitivity can explain all the changes; the original "type 80" strains isolated by ROUNTREE and FREEMAN (1955) were resistant only to penicillin at a time when many strains in hospitals were resistant to several other antibiotics. In 1954, strains of type 80 in Britain and type 80/81 in Canada were resistant to streptomycin and tetracycline as well, but so were many other strains of staphylococci.

It is generally agreed that strains of type 80 (= 80/81) spread in the way that they did because they had a combination of characters that enabled them to colonize hospital patients especially readily. Their ability to produce lesions of the skin, perhaps associated with their lipase activity, has generally been credited with part, at least, of the explanation of their ability. One must postulate that, somehow, a staphylococcus acquired just the right set of characters to enable it to spread, and to produce disease, and that since it had, or acquired, resistance to the most prevalent antibiotics, it was able to initiate the pandemic of the early 1950's.

Staphylococci with the phage pattern 80/81 are not unique in their ability to spread in epidemic fashion. The recent study of LIDWELL and others (1970) illustrates the extensive spread in one hospital ward of staphylococci with the phage pattern 84/85. The potential of this strain for spreading was associated with the fact that it was dispersed far more profusely by carriers than other strains encountered. This spread of the 84/85 strains apparently led to an increased incidence of wound sepsis among patients in the ward.

Changes in phage-type can certainly be associated with other changes in the characters of a staphylococcus. JEVONS and her colleagues (1966) showed that the blocking phages that converted a strain from the typing pattern 83A/84/85 to 84/85 commonly changed the strain's reaction so that the converted strains produced a yellow pigment on glycerol-monoacetate agar and no longer hydrolysed "Tween"; these changes were due to lysogenic conversion. Changes in the carriage of other phages, which may not affect the typing reaction, have also been shown to control the production of the beta-lysin and fibrinolysin.

Moreover, it is now well recognized that phages can transduce antibiotic-resistance-determining genes into staphylococci. BÜLOW (1970) suggested that, in his hospital, the phages leading to the change to the 6557 typing pattern also transduced resistance to neomycin and bacitracin; neomycin resistance has apparently been associated with a plasmid, and is therefore liable to transfer by transduction in some strains other than 84/85. On the other hand JEVONS and co-workers (1966) considered that in the 84/85 strains they examined the neomycin resistance was chromosomal and arose by mutation.

The factors in the staphylococci that determine the observed differences in behaviour and virulence are not known, and there is scope for much more work on various experimental-animal systems as well as study of *in vitro* characteristics. The investigations of AGARWAL (1967) and HILL (1968) on a cell-wall factor that appears to inhibit the inflammatory response, and those of MELISH and GLASGOW (1970) on the ability of some strains to produce characteristic skin lesions, illustrate the directions in which profitable studies might be made, and among such studies must be inquiry into the possibility of introducing virulence factors into relatively innocuous staphylococci by transduction.

Changes in Antibiotic Sensitivity

The "menace of antibiotic resistance in staphylococci" was one of the talking points of the 1950's and appropriately enough when one looks at the reports of the examination of populations of staphylococci isolated from hospital patients between 1946 and 1959 (e.g. MUNCH-PETERSEN and BOUNDY, 1962). It was striking that, in the earlier years, most of the antibiotic-resistant strains were members of phage group III (BARBER and WHITEHEAD, 1949), but with the passage of time, penicillin resistance became widely diffused among strains of all phage groups. At all times, however, a great proportion of the multiple-resistant strains have been members of group III.

The rise in frequency of antibiotic-resistant strains must be largely due to the selection pressure exerted by the widespread use of antibiotics in hospital. It has generally been assumed that selection was operating on the rare mutants that developed resistance independently of exposure to the drugs, but which in the absence of the drugs had no reason to survive (and may even have been penalized in some way in open competition with the sensitive strains). However, the fact that, *in vitro*, antibiotic resistance can certainly be conferred on staphylococci by phage transduction, and the evidence from the study of phage-type distributions already referred to, that phage exchange must take place between staphylococci in the natural environment, indicate that phage-mediated transfer of resistance genes must almost certainly have contributed to the change in resistance pattern. Selection could thus have both mutants and transductants on which to act.

PARKER (in press) has recently drawn attention to an important fact that the selection of strains resistant to one antibiotic is not exercised exclusively by the same antibiotic, and he cites the example of methicillin resistance. Methicillin-resistant strains have increased in frequency with some rapidity in Britain during the last few years (PARKER and HEWITT, 1970) but their frequency does not appear to be related to the use of methicillin in particular hospitals and indeed such strains were isolated in several countries, e.g. Poland, before the introduction of the antibiotic. PARKER postulates that the increase in methicillin-resistant strains in Britain since 1967 is attributable to the great increase in the use of ampicillin; in other countries it may have been high-dosage use of some other penicillin that has acted as the selective agent.

In 1968 BULGER and SHERRIS reported a decline in the proportion of staphylococci resistant to antibiotics in a hospital in Seattle between 1960 and 1967 (Fig. 5). They attributed this partly to the introduction of methicillin, and partly to energetic measures to control cross-infection. RIDLEY and his colleagues (1970) at St. Thomas's Hospital, London, have also reported a decline in the proportion of multiple-resistant staphylococci between 1958 and 1968. They attribute the change in their case largely to an "antibiotic control policy" and discount the effect of measures to combat cross-infection. HEWITT, BROCK and PARKER (pers. communication, 1970) have recently analysed the figures for antibiotic-resistance among staphylococci from several London hospitals. Their figures for St. Mary's Hospital are included in Fig. 5; the decline in the frequency of tetracycline-resistant strains is comparable to that observed by BULGER and SHERRIS and by RIDLEY et al. St. Mary's has not had any formal antibiotic control policy during

this period and measures against cross-infection, though pursued diligently, have
not been nearly as rigorous as those observed in Seattle. There have been great
changes in the phage-types of staphylococci isolated in the hospital, entirely in
line with the national figures shown in Fig. 3.

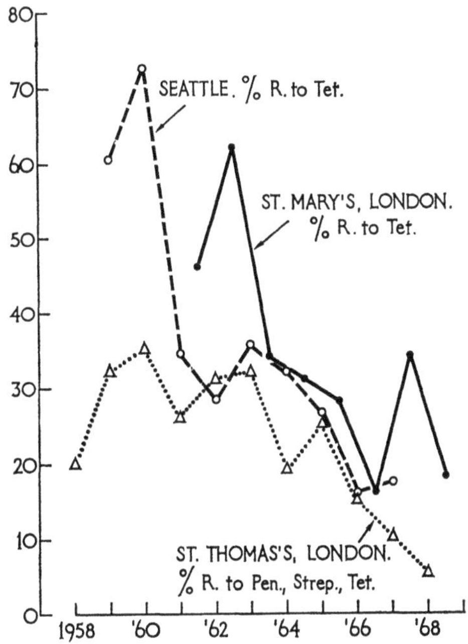

Fig. 5. Changes in prevalence of staphylococci resistant to tetracycline in Seattle (- - - - - BUL-
GER and SHERRIS, 1968) and to penicillin, streptomycin and tetracycline at St. Thomas's
Hospital, London (Δ .... Δ RIDLEY et al., 1970) and St. Mary's Hospital London (————
HEWITT, BROCK and PARKER, pers. communication, 1970)

Conclusion

During the last 30 years the staphylococci in circulation in hospital have undoubtedly changed in phage type and antibiotic sensitivity, and possibly also in
virulence. Although changes in the antibiotics in use in hospitals must have played
a great part in determining these changes, it is difficult to escape the belief that
inherent changes in the staphylococci themselves have also played a great part. It
seems likely that some combination of mutation and lysogenization can, every now
and then, throw up a staphylococcus that has the combination of characters that
are needed for outstanding epidemic propensities.

Presumably the decline of epidemic strains reflects further events of the same
sort. The lysogenization that converted 80/81 to 52/52A/80/81 seems (though
concrete evidence is not really available) to have been associated with a decline in
virulence. If lysogenization can sometimes introduce virulence factors, it must
also sometimes delete them; with time the population of an epidemic type will be

eroded and the strains will revert to "average" staphylococci, or become unrecognizable because of the alteration of type by the acquisition or loss of some phage.

The undoubted powers of spread possessed by the 80/81 staphylococci that were prevalent in the late 1950's must not only have altered the phage-type distribution of hospital staphylococci but must also have impressed the typical 80/81 pattern of antibiotic resistance on the distribution of resistance patterns seen in hospitals. The fact that the staphylococci of the last 8 to 10 years seem, in general, to have less ability to spread means that the nature of the staphylococci themselves may well share, with improved methods of hygiene, the credit for the decline in the prevalence of tetracycline-resistant staphylococci in hospitals, and indeed for other changes.

References

AGARWAL, D. S.: Subcutaneous staphylococcal infection in mice. II. The inflammatory response to different strains of staphylococci and micrococci. Brit. J. exp. Path. 48, 468—482 (1967).

ALDER, V. G., GILLESPIE, W. A.: Influence of neomycin sprays on the spread of resistant staphylococci. Lancet 1967 II, 1062—1063.

ASHESHOV, E. H., RIPPON, J. E.: Changes in typing pattern of phage-type 80 staphylococci. J. gen. Microbiol. 20, 634—643 (1959).

— WINKLER, K. C.: *Staphylococcus aureus* strains in the "52, 52A, 80, 81 complex". Nature (Lond.) 209, 638—639 (1966).

BARBER, M., WHITEHEAD, J. E. M.: Bacteriophage types in penicillin-resistant staphylococcal infection. Brit. med. J. 1949 II, 565—569.

BARNES, B. A., BEHRINGER, G. E., WHEELOCK, F. C., Jr., WILKINS, E. W., Jr.: Surgical sepsis. An analysis of factors associated with sepsis in two operative procedures 1937 to 1957. New Engl. J. Med. 261, 1351—1357 (1959).

— — — — Surgical sepsis: Analysis of factors associated with sepsis following appendectomy (1937—1959). Ann. Surg. 156, 703—712 (1962).

BLAIR, J. E., CARR, M.: Distribution of phage groups of *Staphylococcus aureus* in the years 1927 through 1947. Science 132, 1247—1248 (1960).

BÜLOW, P.: A new epidemic phage type of *Staphylococcus aureus*. 3. Occurrence and spread of "Type 6557", with special reference to the consumption of some antibiotics. Acta path. microbiol. scand. 74, 543—560 (1968).

— A new epidemic phage type of *Staphylococcus aureus*. 5. Epidemic spread of phages among Danish hospital staphylococci. Acta path. microbiol. scand., Sect. B, 78 29—40 (1970).

BULGER, R. J., SHERRIS, J. C.: Decreased incidence of antibiotic resistance among *Staphylococcus aureus*. Ann. intern. Med. 69, 1099—1108 (1968).

FEKETY, F. R., BENNETT, I. L., Jr.: The epidemiological virulence of staphylococci. Yale J. Biol. Med. 32, 23—32 (1959).

HILL, M. J.: A staphylococcal aggressin. J. med. Microbiol. 1, 33—43 (1968).

HOWE, C. W.: Prevention and control of postoperative wound infections owing to *Staphylococcus aureus*. New Engl. J. Med. 255, 787—794 (1956).

JESSEN, O., ROSENDAL, K., BÜLOW, P., FABER, V., ERIKSEN, K. R.: Changing staphylocccoi and staphylococcal infections. New Engl. J. Med. 281, 627—635 (1969).

JEVONS, M. P., JOHN, M., PARKER, M. T.: Cultural characters of a newly recognized group of hospital staphylococci. J. clin. Path. 19, 305—312 (1966).

— PARKER, M. T.: The evolution of new hospital strains of *Staphylococcus aureus*. J. clin. Path. 17, 243—250 (1964).

LIDWELL, O. M., POLAKOFF, S., DAVIES, J., HEWITT, J. H., SHOOTER, R. A., WALKER, K. A., GAYA, H., TAYLOR, G. W.: Nasal acquisition of *Staphylococcus aureus* in a subdivided and mechanically ventilated ward: endemic prevalence of a single strain. J. Hyg. (Lond.) 68, 417—433 (1970).

LINDAU, A., LÖFKVIST, T.: The epidemiology of staphylococcal infections in maternity units. Acta path. microbiol. scand 43, 285—297 (1958).

Lowbury, E. J. L., Babb, J. R., Brown, V. I., Collins, B. J.: Neomycin-resistant *Staphylo coccus aureus* in a burns unit. J. Hyg. (Lond.) **62**, 221—228 (1964).

Melish, M. E., Glasgow, L. A.: The staphylococcal scalded-skin syndrome. Development of an experimental model. New Engl. J. Med. **282**, 1114—1119 (1970).

Munch-Petersen, E., Boundy, C.: Yearly incidence of penicillin-resistant staphylococci in man since 1942. Bull. Wld Hlth Org. **26**, 241—252 (1962).

Parker, M. T., Hewitt, J. H.: Methicillin resistance in *Staphylococcus aureus*. Lancet **1970 I,** 800—804.

Ravenholt, R. T.: History, epidemiology, and control of staphylococcal disease in Seattle. Amer. J. publ. Hlth **52**, 179—809 (1962).

Ridley, M., Barrie, D., Lynn, R., Stead, K. C.: Antibiotic-resistant *Staphylococcus aureus* and hospital antibiotic policies. Lancet **1970 I,** 230—233.

Rountree, P. M.: Changes in the phage-typing patterns of staphylococci following lysogenization. J. gen. Microbiol. **20**, 620—633 (1959).

— Freeman, B. M : Infections caused by a particular phage type of *Staphylococcus aureus.* Med. J. Aust. **2**, 157—161 (1955).

Shooter, R. A., Smith, M. A., Griffiths, J. D., Brown, M. E. A., Williams, R. E. O., Rippon, J. E., Jevons, M. P.: Spread of staphylococci in a surgical ward. Brit. med. J. **1958 I,** 607—613.

Wallmark, G., Finland, M.: Phage types and antibiotic susceptibility of pathogenic staphylococci. Results at Boston City Hospital 1959—1960 and comparison with strains of previous years. J. Amer. med. Ass. **175**, 886—897 (1961).

Williams, R. E. O.: Epidemic staphylococci. Lancet **1959 I,** 190—195.

— Blowers, R., Garrod, L. P., Shooter, R. A.: Hospital infection: causes and prevention, 2nd Ed. London: Lloyd-Luke (Medical Books) Ltd. 1966.

— Rippon, J. E., Dowsett, L. M.: Bacteriophage typing of strains of *Staphylococcus aureus* from various sources. Lancet **1953 I,** 510—514.

Prof. R. E. O. Williams
Department of Bacteriology
Wright-Fleming-Institute
St. Mary's Hospital Medical School
Paddington, London, W. 2. England

Bayer-Symposium III, 111—119 (1971)
© by Springer-Verlag 1971

Pool of Staphylococcal Infections in a Hospital

H. Reber

With 1 Figure

The change of the microbial flora at the site of infection is a problem of ecology. Three conditions must be fulfilled:
1. the presence of a terrain susceptible to be colonized;
2. a bacterial vacuum caused by chemotherapy, and
3. the availability of a secondary invader (Reber).

Clinical observations led to the conclusions, that the first step is an anatomical or functional alteration of a given tissue (e.g. chronic bronchitis) which creates the basic condition for microbial colonisation. The infection constitutes the second step although it is the first to be observed. Only in certain virus diseases (e.g. influenza, rubella) does the infection initiate the events.

This initial anatomical or functional lesion persists despite successful antimicrobial therapy; the latter creates a vacuum which tends to be filled by a new infection, i.e. by a secondary invader. The species of the secondary invader depends on the ecologic circumstances on the one hand and on the antimicrobial barrier produced by antibiotics on the other.

Though all pathogenic bacteria can act as secondary invaders the most frequently found are, in fact, staphylococci, *Pseudomonas* and *Proteus*-species which also have the common properties that they are very rarely primary causative agents, that their nutritional requirements are few, and that they are initially resistant to the common antibiotics or able to develop this property.

The prevalence of staphylococci, *Pseudomonas* and *Proteus* as secondary invaders is conditioned by their relative frequency in the hospital environment. In fact, the great majority of changes in bacterial flora are observed during hospital treatment and must be considered as an important form of hospital infection.

The function of a hospital as a place for care and treatment implies that it constitutes an important pool of infections which entails a considerable risk for all its inhabitants—personnel and patients.

The pool of staphylococcal infections is in no way uniform. It is composed of a multitude of strains, some of which can be distinguished by their lysotype, their antigenic structure, their behaviour toward antibiotics and by their biochemical properties (Baird-Parker).

In the Bürgerspital in Basle, practically every manifest infection is investigated bacteriologically; the isolated staphylococci are phage-typed and tested for susceptibility to antibiotics. We used the official set of bacteriophages issued by the Staphylococcal Reference Laboratory, Colindale, which includes 27 phages subdivided into five groups:

Group	Phages
I	29, 52, 52A, 79, 80
II	3A, 3B, 3C, 55, 71
III	6, 7, 42E, 47, 53, 54, 88, 75, 77, 83A
IV	42D, 1380
Misc	81, 187, 77Ad, D, B5

The phages were propagated by the Bacteriological Laboratory, Bürgerspital, Basle, acting as a national reference laboratory.

For the year 1969, the lysotype most frequently found was 77, B5 (1 RTD); but at 1,000 RTD some other phages of the group III and Misc reacted also, e.g. 7, 47, 54, 75, 77, D, B5. These also were prevalent in 1970.

Table 1. *Lysotypes of* Staphylococcus aureus
(Bürgerspital, Basel 1965)

		%
Total strains	1194	100
Not typable	459	38
Typable with 1 RTD	212	18
Typable with 1,000 RTD	523	44

Table 2. *Lysotypes of* Staphylococcus aureus

Type	Number		Percent		Total
	1 RTD	1,000 RTD	1 RTD	1,000 RTD	
77 Ad	71	125	9.7	17.0	26.7
54	15	28	2.0	3.8	5.8
80	13	20	1.7	2.7	4.5
52	20	6	2.7	0.8	3.5
83 A	12	7	1.6	0.9	2.5

The predominating staphylococcus, the so-called hospital strain, can change in the course of time. In the first years after 1960, 60% of isolated strains were non-typable, more than the average of other laboratories. This changed when the type 77Ad was introduced in the set of phages. In 1965, 1,194 strains of staphylococci were typed, 18% were typable at 1 RTD, 44% at 1,000 RTD. From the typable strains, 26.7% belongs to the phage group 77Ad. This strain must be considered as a so-called hospital strain; in fact, 81% of strains of this type were found in patients who had been in the hospital more than 4 days, and 98.7% were penicillin-resistant as compared with 65% of group I strains (Tables 1 to 4).

Table 3. *Lysotypes of* Staphylococcus aureus. *Susceptibility to penicillin as related to length of hospital stay*

Inhibition zone, mm	4 days or less				5 days and more			
	No.	0—16 %	17—28 %	29 %	No.	0—16 %	17—28 %	29 %
Not typable	105	42	43	15	264	84	10	5
77 Ad	44	95	0	5	189	99.5		0.5
Group I	169	61	28	11	93	74	18	8
Group III	45	57	29	12	84	87	9	4
Misc.	26	58	31	11	47	97		3
	405[a]	59	29	11	681[a]	88.8	7.7	3.5

[a] Incl. group II.

Table 4. *Lysotypes of* Staphylococcus aureus. *Susceptibility to penicillin, oleandomycin and methicillin related to length of hospital stay*

Inhibition zone, mm	4 days or less				5 days and more			
	No.	0—16 %	17—28 %	29 %	No.	0—16 %	17—28 %	29 %
Penicillin								
Not typable	105	42	43	15	264	84	10	5
Typable	300	66	24	10	447	91	6	3
Oleandomycin								
Not typable	105	14	82	4	255	35	64	1
Typable	303	12	87	1	394	26	73.5	0.5
Methicillin								
Not typable	104	15	82	3	255	25	72	3
Typable	303	11	85	3	455	27	71	2

Table 5. *Lysotypes of* Staphylococcus aureus *(Bürgerspital Basel, 1969)*

Phage type			%	%
Not typable		339		40
Typable		507		60
Group III + Misc.	232		46	
Group I	69		13	
Group III	63		12	
Group II	29		6	
Others	114		23	
	507	846	100	100

In 1969, 846 strains of staphylococci were typed from the medical and surgical services. 40% were non typables and of the typables, 46% belong to the type 77, B5 (Table 5).

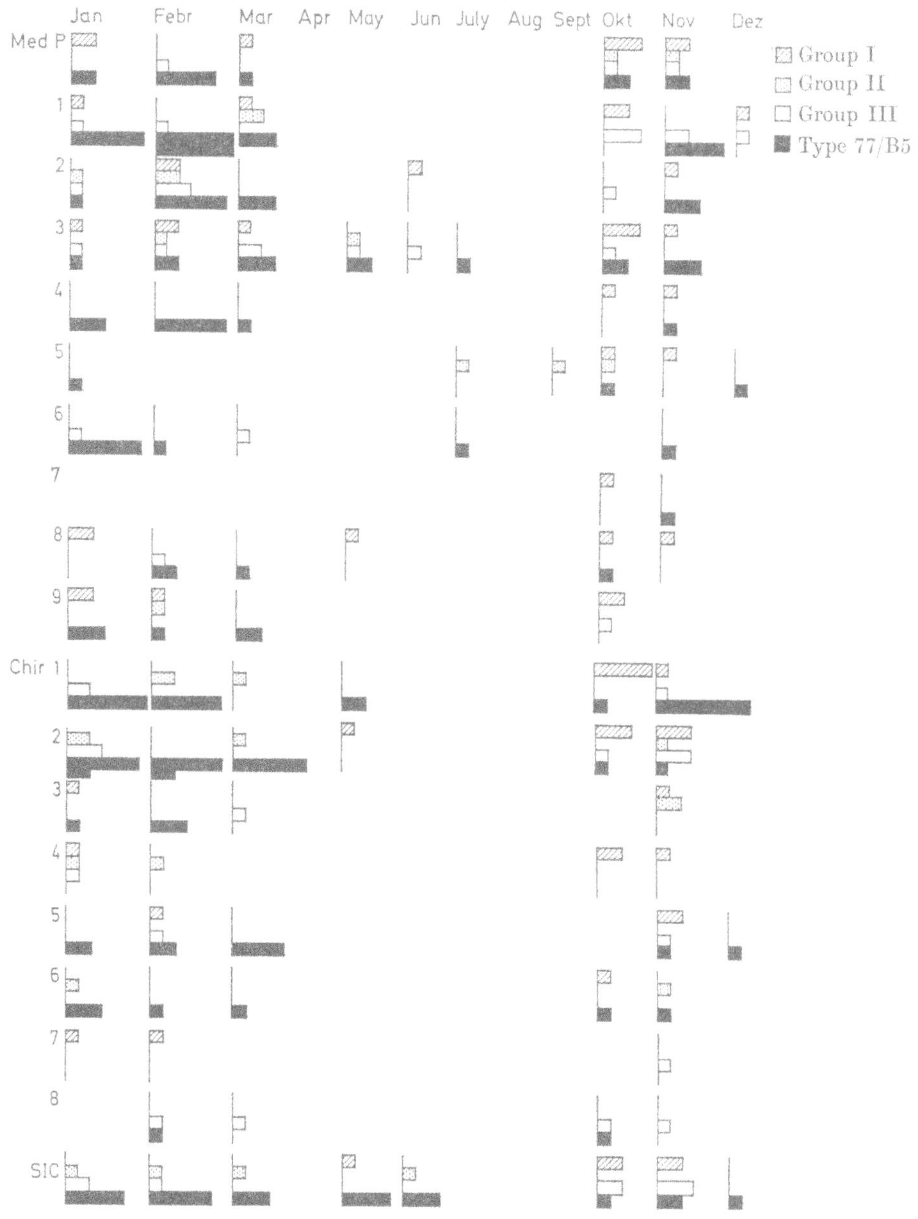

Fig. 1

This observation confirms the well-known fact that the strains of *Staphylococcus aureus* in a given hospital can change over a period of years (PARKER and JEVONS).

The hospital strains seem to present seasonal variations. In the winter their rate is high and in the summer it is lower, returning again in the cold period (Fig. 1).

It is improbable that this variation is an artefact. In the colder periods the diseases susceptible to staphylococcal infections like bronchopneumonia, chronic bronchitis etc., are more frequent. It is highly probable that the spread of staphylococci is favoured in the cold seasons. In the nursery, EICHENWALD described the so-called "cloud baby", and it is probable that this mechanism is also valid for adults.

The hospital strains are irregularly distributed within a hospital.

By analysing the reappearance of staphylococcal infections in the autumn of 1969, between the 1st September and the 31st December,1969, on the basis of the clinical documentation, the following correlations were found (Table 6).

From the 24 lesions with staphylococci of phage group I, 16 were present at the beginning of the hospital stage and were therefore introduced from outside of the hospital. Three cases were acquired in the hospital—having negative

Table 6

Place of Acquisition	Type I	77/B5	
Introduced from outside	16	4	
Certainly acquired in the hospital	3	9	29
Appeared during hospital stay	—	20	
Unknown	5	—	
Total	24	33	

findings at the beginning of their hospital stays, and 5 were uncertain (1 found in feces).

The majority of patients who harboured staphylococci of group I at the beginning of the hospital stay presented some chronic or recurrent illness such as chronic bronchitis, diabetes etc., and had repeated earlier hospital admissions.

A classical example is the group I infection on Medicine 9: the patient harboured it at the time of entry; she was secretary of the head of the obstetrical department of another hospital!

In the transplantation unit, the group I *Staphylococcus aureus* seems to be endemic; three patients were affected.

An analogous example is given by the neurosurgical intensive care station. All three cases appeared in one ward, were comatose and had undergone endotracheal intubation and/or tracheotomy.

The infections with staphylococci of type 75/B5 are different from those with type I. Of the 33 infections due to that type, 9 were acquired in the hospital, being negative upon entry; 20 appeared during the stay in the hospital, and 4 were introduced by patients who had been admitted repeatedly to the Bürgerspital.

In the surgical clinic, the place of acquisition seems to be the surgical intensive care station. Of the 12 surgical cases of type 77/B5 staphylococci, 6 stayed on the surgical intensive care station, 2 certainly acquired the type on this occasion, habouring group I at the time of entry, which later changed to group III. The strain was introduced by a patient with a perianal abscess, who stayed for long periods in the intensive care unit and must be considered as the source of infection.

The strain of Staphylococcus harboured by a given patient can change during the hospital stay. From one patient with renal transplantation, type 80/81 was isolated repeatedly in the fluid of peritoneal dialysis, in the infected bypass, and in the blood. This lysotype persisted the entire year until the 18th June 1970; during the following week this staphylococcal strain was replaced by the hospital strain 77/B5 which had persisted to the present. The exact reason for this change was not discovered; we know only that the patient has had contact with another patient harbouring this lysotype. It is noteworthy that the change took place within the short period of a week, both in the infected bypass, as well as in the peritoneal dialysis fluid. On the one hand, it is accepted as a rule that during the hospital stay the rate of carriers harbouring the hospital strain rises, whereas the infection with a new staphylococcus strain is frequently hindered by a previously established staphylococcal infection. This phenomenon of interference has been used in the prevention of staphylococcal infections in the newborn by inoculating him soon after the birth or after antibiotic treatment. However, a preexisting strain can be overcome with repeated inoculations of heavy doses of non-pathogenic staphylococci (SHINEFIELD et al.).

The data presented illustrate some well-known facts:

1. Staphylococcal infections are not limited to the surgical services or the operation theatre; every speciality can be affected and present its own forms of staphylococcal involvement.

2. Staphylococcal infections in a hospital are a dynamic event. Some strains are introduced; then, depending on the circumstances, the infection either ends abruptly or spreads over the accessible part of a hospital. Furthermore, some strains temporarily or permanently circulate in a hospital. Finally, strains are removed by the departure of the carriers or infected persons from the hospital.

3. The infectious pool in a hospital is a complex one, the distribution of strains varies depending on the time and place. Consequently it is impossible to establish a rule about the frequency of staphylococcal infections applicable for every hospital. The frequency of infections is an individual distinctive mark of a hospital at a given time.

4. In a given patient, the infectious strain can change during his hospital stay, probably as an effect of antibiotic treatment, or by repeated inoculation with heavy doses, or both.

5. From the hospital, the strains can enter in the household and in the population where it is generally dissipated.

Two points should be made about current studies:

1. The observations do not concern the "wild" life of the hospital staphylococcus but a form of hospital epidemic moderated by many preventive measures. Precautions were strictly observed on the surgical intensive care unit. Numerous control studies of the surgical intensive care station have resulted in the failure to isolate typable strains of *Staphylococcus aureus* on the floor, beds, tables and other utensils.

2. The study does not consider the carriers among patients and personnel who played an important role in the transmission of the staphylococci.

The problem is illustrated by the following observation: A patient with staphylococcal septicemia was introduced into the medical intensive care station. Three days later a patient lying obliquely opposite to the first and suffering from a respiratory infection was colonized by the same strain, type 29/52/79/55. The room and personnel were examined systematically. The same Staphylococcus was found in the first patient: on the pillow, the bed linen, the bedside table, the floor under and near the bed and the wall behind the bed near the floor. Approximately the same places were found positive for Staphylococcus in the second patient. The air sampled between 7 and 8 a.m. immediately after making the beds nearby everyone of the four beds located in the room, was also positive but they were negative at noon. Four of the 25 persons of the staff harboured the same type in the nose: 1 of the 3 physicians, the head nurse, 1 maid and 1 physiotherapist. The personnel were released from duty, the patients isolated, and the rooms desinfected by formalin vapour. No manifest infection was observed after that.

The factors that govern the establishment of a staphylococcus strain as a permanent member of a hospital flora are extremely complex.

The hospital strains present a higher infectivity than others. SHOOTER et al. reported the introduction in a ward of a type 79w strain, which colonized the noses of 57 people, caused no sepsis, and disappeared after 3 months.

This high infectivity is frequently, but not always, combined with a higher ability to produce lesions, a higher pathogenicity. FEKETY et al. found that 70% of 49 babies colonized with a given strain suffered clinically manifest infections as compared with 3% of 92 babies colonized with other strains.

Multiple antibiotic resistance, or a corresponding mutation potential, gives a strain a potent selective advantage in competition with others (ROUNTREE).

Finally, the ability of the staphylococci to survive in depots outside the body, in dust, bedding or clothing and to retain its infectivity under these circumstances could be an important factor for the persistence of a strain in the hospital environment (ROUNTREE and GLEN).

The organisation of a modern hospital implies that the infection can spread from certain focal points to different services. Such points are the different intensive care stations where the nature of the care necessitates a closer contact between the patients and where the risk of contamination is, therefore, much higher. The same is true for other areas like central examination wards, radiological services, etc., in which patients are temporarily concentrated. The ambulant specialists, physicians, physiotherapists, laboratory technicians occasionally constitute mobile sources of infection.

The importance of the operating theatre is frequently overestimated. The rigourous discipline governing the staff and the observed asepsis suffice generally to prevent infections. The most dangerous people in this area are the anesthesists, particularly if they visit the patients before or after operations.

Within the hospital, the infection spreads from patients or personnel presenting staphylococcal lesions or carrying staphylococci, and furthermore, from inanimate depots.

The most important dissemination is produced by staphylococcal lesions, like impetigo, bronchopneumonias etc., liberating great quantities of staphylococci. The carriers harbour the staphylococci in the nares and on the perineum. From these sites the microbes reach the adjacent skin and the clothes and are deposited on the fingers. From 19 nasal carriers examined by HARE, 14 harboured the staphylococci on the fingers, 11 on the face, 7 in the hair, 4 on the thorax, 4 on the abdomen and 9 on the clothing.

From the carrier the infection can spread by cross-infection or by autoinfection. In the latter case, the organism is transmitted *per continuitatem* or *per contiguitatem* from the site of carriage on a lesion on the same body.

Cross-infection may recur:

— by air;

— by direct contact;

— by indirect contact via fomites, like handkerchiefs, clothing, bed-linen, soap, instruments, etc.

The spread by droplets seem to be frequently overestimated. Nasal carriers normally disseminate only a few staphylococci around them (ROUNTREE). The minimum dose of 52/52A/80/81 staphylococci to establish 5 day nasal colonisation is large, 10^4 or more organisms. A spread was detected only when levels of 10^3 or more organisms per nasal swab were present for several days (EHRENKRANZ).

But the nasal carrier may be a dangerous spreader when he is suffering from an other respiratory infection. In pediatric wards, the staphylococcal infections spread frequently from babies who suffered from respiratory infections caused by ECHO or adenovirus. Such carriers are surrounded during this affection by a veritable cloud of bacteria ("cloud babies", EICHENWALD) and may infect half of the babies present within 24 h after their entry in a ward.

By antibiotic treatment, innocuous carriers can be converted into dangerous spreaders. EHRENKRANZ demonstrated that tetracycline treatment of carriers with teracycline-resistant *S. aureus* may increase the level of this inapparent infection so that it results in transmission of infection to others. The most important route of transmission is by the fingers, directly or indirectly over fomites.

Dust can act as a heavy depot. Every movement results in a dispersion of staphylococci from the clothing. By improper techniques of bed making, the staphylococci can be dispersed in the air and fall as dust to a distance of 1 to 1.2 m around the bed. Air movements can whirl the dust, which contaminates utensils, instruments and dressings.

In summary, the pool of staphylococci in a hospital is an important source of secondary infection. The behaviour of this pool is very complex and is characterized by a high dynamism and an astonishing adaptability, which transforms the prevention of staphylococcal transmission into a continuous, skillfully conducted battle between the microbiologists and his lovely enemy, the staphylococcus.

References

BAIRD-PARKER, A. C.: A classification of micrococci and staphylococci based on physiological and biochemical tests. J. gen. Microbiol. 30, 409—427 (1963).

DUGUID, J. P., WALLACE, A. T.: Air infection with dust liberated from clothing. Lancet 1948 II, 854.

EHRENKRANZ, N. J.: Transmission of *Staphylococcus aureus* in man — epidemiologic and experimental studies. In: MAIBACH, H. I., HILDICK-SMITH, G.: Skin bacteria and their role in infection, No. 15, p. 201—215. New York: McGraw-Hill 1965.

EICHENWALD, H. F., KOTSEVALOV, O., FASSO, L. A.: The "cloud baby": An example of bacterial-viral interaction. Amer. J. Dis. Child. 100, 161—173 (1960).

FEKETY, F. R., BUCHBINDER, L., SHAFFER, E. I., GOLDBERG, S., PRICE, H. P., PYLE, L. A.: Control of an outbreak of staphylococcal infections among mothers and infants in a suburban hospital. Amer. J. publ. Hlth 48, 298 (1958).

HARE, R.: Dispersal of staphylococci. In: WILLIAMS, R. E. O., SHOOTER, R. A.: Infection in hospitals, p. 75—86. Oxford: Blackwell Scientific Publ. 1963.

PARKER, M. T., JEVONS, M. P.: Hospital strains of staphylococci. In: WILLIAMS, R. E. O., SHOOTER, R. A.: Infection in hospitals, p. 55—65. Oxford: Blackwell Scientific Publ. 1963.

RAVENHOLT, R. T.: Spread of micro-organisms from hospital to community. In: WILLIAMS, R. E. O., SHOOTER, R. A.: Infection in hospitals, p. 179—188. Oxford: Blackwell Scientific Publ. 1963.

REBER, H.: Erregerwechsel als Funktion von Terrain und Chemotherapie. Drug Res. 21, 314—319 (1971).

ROUNTREE, P. M.: Hospital strains of Staphylococcus aureus. In: WILLIAMS, R. E. O., SHOOTER, R. A.: Infection in hospitals, p. 67—73. Oxford: Blackwell Scientific Publ. 1963.

— GLEN, X.: Zit. in: ROUNTREE, P. M.: Hospital strains of Staphylococcus aureus. In: WILLIAMS, R. E. O., SHOOTER, R. A.: Infection in hospitals, p. 72. Oxford: Blackwell Scientific Publ. 1963.

SHINEFELD, H. R., RIBBLE, J. C., EICHENWALD, H. F., BORIS, M., SUTHERLAND, J. M.: Bacterial interference. In: MAIBACH, H. I., HILDICK-SMITH, G.: Skin bacteria and their role in infection, No. 17, p. 235—251. New York: McGraw-Hill 1965.

SHOOTER, R. A., SMITH, M. A., GRIFFITHS, J. D., BROWN, M. E. A., WILLIAMS, R. E. O., RIPPON, J. E., JEVONS, M. P.: Spread of staphylococci in a surgical ward. Brit. med. J. 1958 I, 607.

Prof. Dr. H. REBER
Med. Univ.-Klinik, Bürgerspital
CH-4000 Basel

Discussion

PULVERER: I believe that you have to differentiate clearly among the various potentialities of Staphylococcus aureus, for example, the capacity to multiply and to cause real epidemics. We have seen strains that got into the hospital and caused one severe infection but no more; other strains came in and spread throughout the hospital but caused only a few infections, and then there were the real epidemic strains. Unfortunately, we do not know much about the real reasons for virulence, spreading capacity, or epidemic capacity. I hope, Prof. WILLIAMS, that you agree with me.

WILLIAMS: Yes.

PULVERER: We found some differences in the cell-wall function between epidemic and non-epidemic virulent strains but I do not know if this difference is significant. We have to look more at the functional properties of these features for some answer to this capacity of the staphylococcal strains. Your research has shown that there is something there but it is very difficult to find out what it is. Prof. REBER mentioned "interference" of Staphylococcus albus. The latest results reported at Atlanta (from the Communicable Disease Center or the U.S. Public

Health Service) and others which indicate that it may be quite dangerous to use interference (with strain 502). These are very good examples.

KASS: I would like to see if we can at least try to define some of these concepts in operational terms which might help us to set up the experiments to get at some of the problems. In the intestinal tract, we know, from studies in volunteers, that the implantation of a pathogen into the intestinal tract is largely a matter of the size of inoculum administered. If the inoculum is small, no isolations occur from the feces, but as the inoculum increases there are more and more positive isolations of organisms such as Salmonella. Do we have any evidence that it is different with Staphylococcus? How much of the pattern that we are seeing represents no more than the numbers available to the site in which the organisms were planted?

If numbers alone are the major determinant, then the question of relative virulence of strains becomes secondary. I am not yet certain that we have seen good evidence that strains vary that much in virulence. We have not yet separated the factor of numbers of organisms from the question of intrinsic virulence, as a quality peculiar to any single micro-organism. Do we have evidence that transduction per se is a powerful factor? The rate at which transduction operates to produce a new strain with given characteristics is in the order of $1/10^{7-8}$. Therefore, selection pressures would need to be intense in order to cause one strain to become dominant after transduction.

Has anyone any insight into the precise factors, other than antibiotic usage, that might influence the accumulation of a larger number of any given strain after transduction? It seems to me that the problem could be looked upon as a purely quantitative one, and, if so, we would then want to pay more attention to the question of what brings large numbers of organisms into a community and into contact with the individual, rather than being so concerned with the precise way in which the original mutational change occurred.

WILLIAMS: I think there is an answer to Prof. KASS's first question, that is, whether the whole pattern, or a large part, can be explained by simple differences in dose (inoculum). Dr. LIDWELL has done some very nice analyses relating the dose of staphylococci probably inhaled by patients in hospital wards, to the acquisition of nasal carriage. He showed that there is a dose-response relationship. He also showed that the relationship is different for tetracycline-resistance staphylococci from what it is for tetracycline-sensitive strains; the tetracycline-resistant strains are established more easily than the tetracycline-sensitive strains for a given dose of the organisms. So I am sure that the dose to which the patient is exposed is a very important factor in determining whether he becomes a nasal carrier of Staphylococcus, but I am equally sure it is by no means a sufficient explanation for all the observed phenomena.

We monitored the air of a small hospital ward for over a year on a 24 h basis and showed very clearly that active dispersers of staphylococci, who raised the air count in the ward to 20 or 30 times its base-level, were not uncommon, but it was on only a very small proportion of the occasions, when an active disperser was introduced, that other patients acquired the staphylococci. This certainly seemed to be quite clearly associated with particular staphylococci.

KASS: Could that not possibly be a function of numbers with the active dispersers, simply making more bacteria available for implantation?

WILLIAMS: No, I do not think so, there were plenty of active dispersers of strains which did not establish themselves in other people.

KASS: Again the problem is that there are two variables operating: the number of organisms discharged or available to the patient and the specific selection circumstances. Could it not be that the problem is simply one of numbers of organisms available to colonize a patient?

WILLIAMS: Yes, I would have thought that it was. I would have thought that the whole patternof the epidemiology of staphylococci in the hospital would deny your thesis that the differences could be explained solely in terms of numbers, though I am sure that numbers are very important.

I would like to take up one of the other points—one that Prof. PULVERER mentioned too. I am sure that we have to look for other characteristics in staphylococci that may not be of particular taxonomic value but which are of "aggressive" value to the staphylococcus. My colleagues found an aggressive factor in cell walls of staphylococci which appears to be anti-inflammatory and which enables staphylococci to establish themselves more readily in the tissues—at least in the skin of the mouse. We have to follow this up in a variety of ways. We need to discover whether the same factor is relevant to virulence in man and, of course, it would also be interesting to see whether this is a characteristic which can be transduced by phages.

SHOOTER: It would be interesting and valuable to know if staphylococci retain their ability to infect long after they have been shed from the patient? Some years ago, PHYLISS ROWNTREE suggested that this was a possible attribute of dangerous staphylococci.   We were interested at the time because we had followed the records of a thousand patients who had been nursed in woolen blankets, which were not often disinfected; with one doubtful exception, we found no example of a patient who acquired a staphylococcus of the same type from the previous occupant of the bed.

I am still waiting to have my view shaken that once the staphylococcus has been shed for 24 h, it is unlikely to infect another person. As a rider to that, Prof. PULVERER, would you agree perhaps with the experience that Prof. WILLIAMS and I had, that it is rash to talk about patients coming in and spreading infection without qualification, because in our extensive records, nearly all the patients who came in and spread infection were those carrying tetracycline-resistant staphylococci. We were observing patients at the time in open wards and we found practically no example of spread starting from patients with boils or carbuncles when the infecting staphylococcus was sensitive to tetracycline.

PULVERER: I agree with you.

FINLAND: I recall the days before sulfonamides when ALVIN COBURN reported a series of studies on the spread of streptococcal infections in a home for rheumatic children. That was after the introduction of the Griffith types and he followed the introduction and spread of various serotypes of streptococci *seriatim* into the ward.

As I recall, any new strain that was introduced usually colonized the great majority of children but generally did not produce any infections as evidenced by pharyngitis, or other signs of disease, or by an increase in antistreptolysin titre in the serum, and this was not followed by recrudescences of rheumatic fever. However, on certain occasions a new type would be introduced and would invariably produce a high percentage of actual infection among those children and these were generally followed by some recrudescences of rheumatic fever in those children. Sometimes one type would occur—would go through a ward and not produce disease and on another occasion that type would produce infections and theumatic fever. I think he used the term "invasiveness" to describe this character of the streptococcus, he did not identify it other than by its pathogenicity because is was not limited to any specific type of Streptococcus.

With respect to Prof. SHOOTER's remark about the loss of virulence, once a strain is shed. I can recall during the World War II there were intensive studies of streptococcal disease in the U.S. Army at Camp Clayburn and Fort Warren and elsewhere. The dust from the wards assigned to patients with acute streptococcal infections was collected, resuspended and inoculated directly into the nasopharynx of normal volunteers. This failed to produce disease with the same types of streptococci as those infecting the patient. On the other hand, direct nasopharyngeal secretions from infected patients to normal volunteers regularly produced the disease. It was a sort of an heroic experiment, but I think it brought out this point about virulence; although these organisms could be grown in culture from the dust, they could not establish themselves in volunteers even when massive numbers were inoculated. In these experiments the dose of streptococci from dust and from secretion of infected patients was quantitatively the same by colony counts.

WILLIAMS: I would like to follow this up because this is certainly an area where Prof. KASS's remarks on dosage are very important. If you have a chain of ten streptococci, 90% can die before the viable count changes, as determined by the bacteriologist, and in the drying of clumps of staphylococci the same thing can happen. Before we can say that an organism loses it virulence on drying, we must take great care that the dose that we are giving is really the same and not just spuriously the same as a result of the inefficiency of ordinary viable counting. In work that we have done with subcutaneous infections of staphylococci in mice, we were unable to detect a difference between dried and fresh cocci provided the numbers of viable cells were the same.

KASS: This was exactly the point I was going to make in response to some of the experiments that have been cited. One can use Waring blenders to break up chains or clusters and show that the ratio of live to dead cells changes very strikingly with time, although the apparent number of colony forming units in the original suspension does not change very much. This is a critical point in studying this problem.

SHOOTER: I am sure that numbers are involved in determining how long the staphylococcus is going to cause damage after it has been shed. But you do have quite clear examples of outbreaks which are very difficult to link with numbers only. Some years ago, we had a ward where a nurse came back with a septic lesion on her hand. This was at a time when there had been no record of epidemic sepsis due to type 80/81 staphylococci for several years. Within 10 days we had twelve nurses with septic lesions on the hand due to characteristic 80/81 strains and six patients also became infected. I think it is difficult not to accept this idea that this strain 80/81 has special properties and I doubt if an explanation, based solely on extra numbers, fits all the facts.

KASS: I will accept the possibility, but I hope you will accept with me the equal possibility that what the nurse did was to introduce a larger number of viable staphylococci that were now available for dissemination, when prior to that the available number of viable 80/81 staphylococci were exceedingly low. There may be simple explanations or complex ones but the trouble with studying problems of virulence in staphylococci is that this has been going on for almost 10 years and we have not succeeded in finding very much that is valuable. I prefer to give up on problems when no one has found anything that is useful.

Bayer-Symposium III, 125—130 (1971)

Changes of the Infectious Pool in the Hospital with Regard to *Pseudomonas aeruginosa* and *Escherichia coli*

R. A. SHOOTER

There seems to be agreement from most centres that in recent years there has been an increase in the incidence of infections due to gram-negative bacilli. It would be easy to document this with references to special situations such as the prevalence of *Pseudomonas aeruginosa* in burns units, or to the frequency of isolation of intestinal gram-negative bacilli from blood cultures in patients after surgery. But this would be a statement of recorded findings and say little about the source of the organisms themselves. If we want to know where they come from, we are probably going to be restricted to those organisms for which typing methods are available. In this paper I would like to discuss the situation in regard to *Ps. aeruginosa* and *Escherichia coli*. As typing has not yet been used extensively for epidemiological purposes, discussion will have to be confined to the present position rather than to a comparison between the position now and in the past.

Ps. aeruginosa

Ps. aeruginosa is a hardy organism, that needs little nutrient for growth and is difficult to kill with antibiotics and with many disinfectants. It is not easy to be sure why it is more prominent now than it was in the past. In part it probably reflects the ability to treat and eradicate other organisms from infections, leaving *Ps. aeruginosa* still there as a more difficult treatment problem. Older patients, longer operations and various forms of therapy may have produced more susceptible patients, and there is the possibility that selection, particularly in hospital, has produced strains of Pseudomonas with a greater capacity to cause damage than those present previously.

It is not always clear if Pseudomonas is acting as a pathogen when it is isolated from patients, but in a number of situations there is no doubt that it is. In the eye it has been responsible for many disasters and it is a well recognised pathogen in burns and in infections of the urinary tract. In skin wounds and ulcers it may merely be present as a colonist, but in some cases it delays healing and it can be the reason for the failure of grafts to take. It is a cause of meningitis, septicaemia and rarely of endocarditis. Its role in the chest is more equivocal. Although a common isolate from tracheostomies, and found perhaps with increasing frequency in the sputum of patients in intensive care units, it seems that it is not often the primary pathogen responsible for respiratory infection.

We still have much more to discover about the source of Pseudomonas in the patient's environment and the way in which patients are infected, but much is already known.

Burns

Patients with burns fall in a special category. Once the burns are infected, enormous numbers of bacteria may be shed, and as it is often the practice to treat burnt patients together in units, other patients may be infected very rapidly. There is some evidence to suggest that patients treated in isolation or in wards with patients without burns are less likely to acquire infection.

Medicaments

Because of its ability to grow easily and its resistance, *Pseudomonas aeruginosa* has been found in many lotions, medicaments and disinfectants (Lowbury, 1951; Plotkin and Austrian, 1958; Lee and Failkow, 1961; Phillips, 1966; Noble and Savin, 1966). Much, if not all, of this form of contamination can be prevented without undue effort. Corks—themselves difficult to sterilise—contribute sufficient nutriment to lotions in bottles for the growth of Pseudomonas, and by now one should no longer find disinfectant and lotion bottles with cork stoppers (Anderson and Keynes, 1958; Nelson, 1942). They should be supplied in small quantities, preferably in dated containers, and, where possible, sterilised after preparation. For some things, such as eye drops, single dose preparations should be used. The source of contamination varies. It has been traced, among other sources, to a number of unsterile practices in the pharmacy and to the water used in dispensing.

Respirators and Incubators

Respirators and incubators have commonly been involved in the infection of patients (Laursen, 1963; Barrie, 1965; Bassett et al., 1965; Phillips and Spencer, 1965; Rubbo et al., 1966). Until recently little thought has been given by their designers to the need to construct them in such a way that disinfection is possible. Ideally, perhaps, they should be able to stand sterilisation by heat, or to have the parts concerned disposable. Meanwhile with many of the existing machines, the patient has to be protected by the use of filters, keeping the humidifier, if fitted, at 60 °C, and by disinfection of the apparatus after use with ethylene oxide gas or liquid chemical disinfectants.

Cystoscopes, Catheters and Urine Drainage Systems

In the past, failure to sterilise cystoscopes and catheters and the use of open drainage systems for patients with indwelling catheters led to many urinary infections. These should not now occur with proper sterilisation and closed drainage, although in the nursing and treatment of patients with infected urine careful asepsis is essential, as infected urine is an excellent potential source of further infections (Macleod, 1958; Pyrah et al., 1955; Gillespie et al., 1964; Roberts et al., 1965).

General Considerations

In most hospitals outbreaks of infection with Pseudomonas occur only rarely, 1. at all. The pattern is more often of sporadic infection, isolated cases appearing in scattered parts of the hospital. Some of these infections are probably examples of direct cross-infection from one patient to another. Except in unusual circumstances, for instances in burns and chest infections, it is unlikely that spread is through the air, and it is more probable that it is a form of contact transfer. With the growing scientific content of the syllabus for both medical and nursing students, there is a tendency to lay less stress on teaching the relatively simple techniques needed for aseptic procedures in the wards. But germs remain with us, and it is still very necessary to train young men and women in the ways in which their spread can be prevented.

Reference has been made to contamination of water by Pseudomonas. This may come from the tank, from the pipes running from the tank to the tap or from the tap, particularly if it is fitted with a rubber and metal nozzle designed to stop splashing or to allow the addition of graded doses of detergent. The waste pipes of baths and basins are difficult to rid of Pseudomonas and have probably been the source of infection in adult patients. In one account, newborn babies were shown to have acquired their Pseudomonas from bathing in a poorly designed and difficult to disinfect basin (COKE et al., 1970). In an indirect way water may have been the source of infection in the interesting series of infections in a neurosurgical unit that were eventually traced to the shaving brush used by the barber when preparing patients for operation (AYLIFFE et al., 1965).

When all extraneous sources are considered, however, there is a strong presumption that many of the infections seen in hospital are autogenous, in that the infecting organisms has come from the patient's own bowel (DARRELL and WAHBA, 1964; SHOOTER et al., 1966).

Autogenous Infection with *Ps. aeruginosa*

Surveys would suggest that about 5% of healthy young adults carry *Ps. aeruginosa* in their bowels. Within some hospitals, at least, the carriage rate is higher, and cumulative rates as high as 40% may be seen, although the reasons for this are not entirely clear. Pseudomonas is found in the majority of patients with ileostomies, and it appears that some antibiotics (GAYA et al., 1970), appear to encourage the proliferation of Pseudomonas in the bowel flora. At one time it was thought that Pseudomonas spread from one patient to another, but in some of the situations that have been investigated it is clear that the organism is swallowed in food or drugs supplied by the hospital (SHOOTER et al., 1969). Improperly disinfected mixing machines used in the preparation of fortified milk feeds have been identified as a reason for contaminated foods. Until recently little attention has been paid to the bacterial content of medicines intended to be swallowed, but these, too, have been shown to transmit Pseudomonas to the patient.

There is now good epidemiological evidence that in some cases the Pseudomonas responsible for clinical infection has come from the patient. In some respects this is an encouraging finding. If not more than 1 patient in 20 is admitted to hospital carrying *Ps. aeruginosa* it should be possible to stop his strain spreading and to ensure that the remaining patients do not acquire Pseudomonas during their stay. It will entail the observation of parts of the hospital such as kitchens and pharmacies that have so far largely escaped the attention of the epidemiologically interested hospital bacteriologist, but with new techniques available, the task should not be too formidable.

Escherichia coli

A somewhat oversimplified statement of the position of *E. coli* current until recently might be that it was a normal bowel inhabitant, albeit constituting only a small proportion of the bowel flora, that with the exception of some special serotypes that caused diarrhoea in very young children it did no damage within the gut, and that once strains of *E. coli* were established there they tended to remain without change for long periods. There are reasons for doubting some of these assumptions. My colleagues and I have been interested in the subject and I would like to discuss it on a speculative basis, well aware that our opinions lack full confirmation and may be applicable only to a special situation.

We became interested some years ago when in the course of a survey over 20 months, of women with chronic urinary tract infections, we found that small groups of patients were infected at the same period with identical serotypes of *E. coli* (SPENCER et al., 1968). As the women were not catheterised or subjected to instrumentation, the patient's own bowel seemed the most probable source of *E. coli*, and the mouth the route by which *E. coli* reached the bowel. Subsequent investigation showed that the faecal *E. coli* flora of female patients in one ward of the same hospital was constantly changing, and that the most likely source of the new strains was the hospital food (COOKE et al., 1969; COOKE et al., 1970). The situation in this hospital was perhaps exceptional in that owing to unhygienic washing up practices in the kitchen, strains of *E. coli* entering the hospital on meat and poultry were recontaminating food after its cooking or during its preparation (SHOOTER et al., 1970).

These findings may be unique. If they are not, they open up several interesting possibilities. Working with a limited range of O typing sera we found that almost all the serotypes we isolated from patients' stools could be isolated from cows and chickens after they were killed. It may be that with a greater range of O sera and with H and K sera it would be possible to show differences between animal and human strains, but at the moment it seems permissible to speculate that although many serotypes of *E. coli* belong primarily to animals and do not establish themselves in humans, some serotypes survive well in both animals and humans. The 27 O sera we used allowed us to type about three quarters of the strains of *E. coli* isolated from patient's stools, and these strains included those commonly responsible for urinary infection.

If this transfer of *E. coli* between animals and man is confirmed and shown to occur in other places, it would give force to those who wish to restrict the use of antibiotics in animal feeding stuffs. It is probable that the chances of transfer of *E. coli* from meat and poultry to food may be greater in institutions than in the home, and this possibility might account for the variations in incidence of O types of *E. coli* causing infections that have been reported in surveys.

Note on the Constancy of the Bowel Flora

Examination of the bowel flora is technically exacting. Even with organisms such as *Ps. aeruginosa* and *E. coli* that grow easily on culture, one can only examine a small sample of the total. For this reason, perhaps, there are conflicting opinions on the constancy of the bowel flora. One school holds that the normal bowel contains a wide range of strains, and that those predominant in the faecal specimen are so by chance, or by some alteration of the internal economy of the bowel. Our present view is that this is unlikely, that relatively few strains are carried at the same time and that the bowel flora is recruited at shorter or longer intervals from organisms swallowed in food and drink. Some support for this was from the work of Dr. STOODLEY (pers. communication) who in 100 consecutive autopsies examined 4 different intestinal sites for *Ps. aeruginosa* and from the finding that *Ps. aeruginosa* (BUCK and COOKE, 1969) and *E. coli* taken by mouth in doses of 10^4 or more organisms would establish themselves in the bowels of volunteers.

References

ANDERSON, K., KEYNES, R.: Infected cork closures and the apparent survival of organisms in antiseptic solutions. Brit. med. J. 1958 II, 272.

AYLIFFE, G. A. J., LOWBURY, E. J. L., HAMILTON, J. G., SMALL, J. M., ASHESHOV, E. A., PARKER, M. T.: Hospital infection with *Pseudomonas aeruginosa* in neurosurgery. Lancet 1965 II, 365.

BARRIE, D.: Incubator-borne *Pseudomonas aeruginosa* infection in a newborn nursery. Arch. Dis. Childh., 40, 555 (1965).

BASSETT, D. C. J., THOMPSON, S. A. S., PAGE, B.: Neonatal infections with *Pseudomonas aeruginosa* associated with contaminated resuscitation equipment. Lancet 1965 I, 781.

BUCK, A. C., COOKE, E. M.: The fate of ingested Pseudomonas in normal volunteers. J. med. Microbiol. 2, 521 (1969).

COOKE, E. M., EWINS, S. P., SHOOTER, R. A.: Changing faecal population of *Escherichia coli* in hospital medical patients. Brit. med. J. 1969 II, 593.

— SHOOTER, R. A., KUMAR, P. J., ROUSSEAU, S. A., FOULKES, A. L.: Hospital food as a possible source of *Escherichia coli* in hospital medical patients. Lancet 1970 I, 436.

— — O'FARRELL, S., MARTIN, D.: Faecal carriage of *Pseudomonas aeruginosa* in newborn babies. Lancet 1970 II, 1045.

DARRELL, J. H., WAHBA, A. H.: Pyocine-typing of hospital strains of *Pseudomonas pyocyanea*. J. clin. Path. 17, 236 (1964).

GAYA, H., ADNITT, P. I., TURNER, P.: Changes in gut flora after cephalexin treatment. Brit. med. J. 1970 II, 624.

GILLESPIE, W. A., LEMMON, G. G., LINTON, K. B., SLADE, N.: Prevention of urinary infection in gynaecology. Brit. med. J. 1964 II, 423.

LAURSEN, H.: Bacteriological colonisation of infants and mothers in a maternity unit. Acta obstet. genec. scand. 42, 43 (1963).

LEE, J. C., FAILKOW, P. J.: Benzalkonium chloride — source of hospital infection with gram-negative bacteria. J. Amer. med. Ass. 177, 708 (1961).

LOWBURY, E. J. L.: Contamination of cetrimide (cetyltrimethylammonium bromide) and other fluids with *Pseudomonas pyocyanea*. Brit. J. industr. Med. 8, 22 (1951).

MACLEOD, J. W.: The hospital urine bottle and bedpan as reservoirs of infection by *Pseudomonas pyocyanea*. Lancet 1958 I, 394.

MITCHELL, J. P., GILLESPIE, W. A.: Bacteriological complications from the use of urethral instruments: Principles of prevention. J. clin. Path. 17, 492 (1964).

NELSON, J. H.: The growth of coliform bacilli in water containing various organic materials. J. Path. Bact. 54, 445 (1942).

NOBLE, W. C., SAVIN, G. A.: Steroid cream contamined with *Pseudonomas aeruginosa*. Lancet 1966 I, 347.

PHILLIPS, I.: Postoperative respiratory tract infection with *Pseudonomas aeruginosa*. Lancet 1966 I, 903.

— SPENCER, G.: *Pseudomonas aeruginosa* cross-infection due to contaminated respiratory apparatus. Lancet 1965 I, 903.

PLOTKIN, S. A., AUSTRIAN, R.: Bacteremia caused by Pseudomonas sp. following the use of materials stored in solutions of a cationic surface active agent. Amer. J. med. Sci. 235, 621 (1958).

Pyrah, L. N., Goldie, W., Parson, F. M., Raper, F. P.: Control of *Pseudomonas pyocyanea* infection in a urological ward. Lancet 1955 II, 314.

Roberts, J. B. M., Linton, K. B., Pollard, B. R., Mitchell, J. P., Gilleseie, W. A.: Long-term catheter drainage in the male. Brit. J. Urol., **37**, 63 (1965).

Rubbo, S. D., Gardner, J. F., Franklin, J. C.: Source of *Pseudomonas aeruginosa* infection in premature infants. J. Hyg. (Lond.) **64**, 121 (1966).

Shooter, R. A., Cooke, E. M., Rousseau, S. A., Breaden, A. L.: Animal sources of common serotypes of *Escherichia coli* in the food of hospital patients. Lancet 1970 II, 226.

— Gaya, Cooke, E. M., Kumar, P., Patel, N., Parker, M. T., Thom, B. T., France, D. R.: Food and medicaments as possible sources of hospital strains of *Pseudomonas aeruginosa*. Lancet 1969 I, 1227.

— Walker, K. A., Williams, V. R., Horgan, G. M., Parker, M. T., Asheshov, E. H., Bullimore, J. F.: Faecal carriage of *Pseudomonas aeruginosa* in hospital patients. Lancet 1966 II, 1331.

Spencer, A. G., Mulcahy, D., Shooter, R. A., O'Grady, F. W., Bettleheim, K. A., Taylor, J.: *Escherichia coli* serotypes in urinary tract infection in a medical ward. Lancet 1968 II, 839.

Prof. R. A. Shooter
Department of Bacteriology
St. Bartholomew's Hospital
London, E.C. 1. England

Discussion

Gould: May I ask Prof. Shooter what numbers of Pseudomonas he isolates from the stools of patients coming into hospital and if, in addition to the increase in incidence of isolation, there is also an average numerical increase amongst those who have become colonized during their stay in hospital? This incidence of 5% amongst the patients that are admitted, I would agree with, particularly if one looks for small numbers of Pseudomonas in the bowel contents, that is less than 10^5/g. In this context there is perhaps a significant change over the last 20 years since in the early 1950's, Macleod and I looked specifically for Pseudomonas in the stools of patients in general practice and also amongst healthy students who had not started their clinical years; we failed to find anyone from whom we could isolate *Pseudomonas aeruginosa*. It would appear, unfortunately not on the basis of having examined exactly the same type of population, that this situation has changed in these 20 years and that, as Prof. Shooter says, there are now a larger number of persons who are carrying this organism in the stool.

Shooter: I do not have with me the numbers, although some are high. Dr. Parker asked me to tell you that one answer to your letter in the Lancet is that the numbers are high. The figures I have given are "all or nothing" answers. One difficulty we have had in this is that our feeding experiments, which Dr. Buck and Dr. Cooke reported, suggested that if you feed a new strain, it may get through in 16 h and it can leave in about 48 h. There is, therefore, some difficulty in deciding what is an "admission" stool. I think if I were going to do this again, I would ask the patient to come to hospital with a specimen of stool.

KASS: Quite contrary to what you may be thinking, I am in complete agreement with you. The experiments on the implantation of a new flora in the bowel are among the few that are quantitatively acceptable. Given the usual bowel flora, competitive factors, probably organic acids produced by the genus *Bacteroides* are such that it takes a large oral inoculum to identify even the so-called pathogens such as typhoid bacilli, other Salmonella etc., in the stool.

I am confident that a minority of the flora will be eliminated very rapidly from the feces unless there is continuous refeeding. Probably the best data that deals with this are those on lactobacilli. If one feeds 10^9 to 10^{11} lactobacilli, there is minimal implantation. If one feeds the same number of these organisms with lactose or lactulose, the implantation is established more rapidly because the lactic acid acts as a microbiological barrier. But even then, unless these organisms and/or substrate are continually refed, so that bacteria will multiply, they disappear quickly.

SHOOTER: Our experience with Pseudomonas bears this out. For establishment, 10^5 or more organisms were needed. In our small numbers of volunteers, the strain was eliminated rapidly, with one exception, a patient who was taking ampicillin and who carried it for a long time. There was also some indication that our patients, under treatment with some antibiotics, tend to carry Pseudomonas longer. I am not quite sure that is going to follow with our feeding experiments with *E. coli*. We do not have many people involved. Some of them are carrying the strain for weeks and in 1 or 2 cases, several months after feeding.

KASS: If one examines the literature on Lactobacillus, it looks as though the one determinant above all others is the availability of a substrate as a source of carbohydrate in the lower bowel. What is suggested here is that there may be specific factors that will permit the selective emergence of one or another organism depending upon its specific nutritive requirements. The well-known experiment of MILLER and HAMMON that has been reproduced repeatedly, namely, that if the microbial content of the flora in the bowel is sufficiently reduced by any sort of external means, such as an antibiotic, then implantation is very much easier to establish. One hundred Salmonella were successfully implanted in mice that had been previously treated with oral streptomycin, whereas it required feeding many millions of organisms before any implantation without the antibiotic was successful.

SHOOTER: You will probably agree that this happens in newborn babies, where it is inconceivable that they get the dosage required in adults.

KASS: I have studied this problem of newborn babies. My conviction, for whatever it is worth, is that a major reason why breast-fed babies have less diarrhoea than the bottle-fed ones is because the breast-fed baby has a lacto-bacillus flora, already present, which acts as a reasonable barrier against the implantation of coliforms and other gram-negative pathogens. We have treated babies with staphylococci replacement of the bowel flora by simply feeding them breast milk and the flora of their stools converted to a lactobacillus flora which replaced the staphylococci completely without the use of antimicrobial agents. In the newborn baby, perhaps the bowel, being empty, is colonized by whatever comes in first; the selective pressures within the bowel are those that are largely dominated by the food intake.

MARGET: In this connexion, I made an observation which was published about 3 years ago. We have seen with premature newborns, 70, 80 or 90% *Pseudomonas aeruginosa* without symptoms, while other newborns, given the same food, have several diseases with nearly the same percentage of the organisms. In normal newborns we have seen about 3 to 5% *Pseudomonas aeruginosa* in the bowel.

VON GRAEVENITZ: I would like to ask Prof. SHOOTER whether he thinks one should do something about *Pseudomonas aeruginosa*, which we have seen in a large percentage of hospital sinks? The drains, in particular, carry this organism.

SHOOTER: There are plenty of people who think one should do something about the sinks. I suspect that this needs investigation in each circumstance. I have little evidence to suppose that in an ordinary surgical ward, Pseudomonas in the sink is necessarily related to illness in the patient. Whether the bath is related may be different. We have a paper, which the Lancet is about to publish, describing an experience in which babies were bathed and acquired Pseudomonas. By either not bathing the babies, or by bathing them in sterile water, we were able to keep free from Pseudomonas.

PULVERER: We studied what could be the relationship between *Pseudomonas aeruginosa* in hospitals and the rising use of synthetic material. We hoped to find some relationship. We received the most important synthetic materials from Bayer in Germany but we could not find that *Pseudomonas aeruginosa* is able to take carbon or nitrogen from synthetic material for metabolism.

Bayer-Symposium III, 133—142 (1971)

Occurrence of *Serratia marcescens* in Soft Tissue Infections

A. von Graevenitz and D. Buchholz

The shift of focus from gram-positive to gram-negative bacteria as agents of nosocomial disease has led to a surge of interest in gram-negative rods that were once assumed to be nonpathogenic, such as species of the genera *Pseudomonas*, *Aeromonas*, *Flavobacterium*, *Actinobacter*, and, in particular, *Serratia*. Between 1894 and 1960, approximately 30 papers on *Serratia* infections appeared in the world literature, while in the past 10 years, 75 papers have covered the subject—not counting those that primarily dealt with in-vitro sensitivities of this organism.

Serratia marcescens is the only species in the genus *Serratia*, family *Enterobacteriaceae*. Its recognition may be difficult if the red pigment, prodigiosin, is not formed on routine media—as is now the case in the overwhelming majority of strains. On "enteric" plates, lactose is not fermented. Dextrose and sucrose, but not arabinose, are fermented with little or no gas formation. H_2S and indol are not formed. Flagella, lysine and ornithine decarboxylase, deoxyribonuclease, and gelatinase are present, and citrate is utilized. The Voges-Proskauer reaction is positive except in the subspecies *kiliensis*.

S. marcescens is widely distributed in nature and has by now become a frequent inhabitant of hospital wards. It may colonize or infect patients with compromised local or general defense mechanisms. Typical transmission occurs in hospital through inhalation therapy equipment, urinary catheters and other instruments, and solutions; data on the carrier state are not available. The organism is resistant to many antimicrobials. At this time, gentamicin, nalidixic acid, and kanamycin/neomycin are the most effective agents in vitro and in vivo (reviews: Clayton and von Graevenitz; Ewing et al.; Fields et al.; von Graevenitz, 1964; Wilfert et al., 1968, 1970).

Most frequently, *S. marcescens* has been isolated from the urinary and respiratory tract and from blood, occasionally from other sources. A few soft tissue infections have been reported, as early as 1894 (du Bois St-Sévrin) and again since 1962 (Bodey et al., Cabrera, Clayton and von Graevenitz, Conn et al., Fields et al., Gale and Sonnenwirth, Magnuson and Elston, Sanders et al., Wilfert et al., 1970), but systematic data on these kinds of infections are lacking.

Material and Methods

Records of the Bacteriology Laboratory—which receives only specimens from patients over 15 years of age—were reviewed for the period between November 1, 1968 and August 31, 1970. 109,500 specimens were received; 2% of them originated from obviously infected soft tissues, i.e., infected wounds and cutaneous or subcutaneous suppurative lesions (not counting lesions from internal organs, from the meninges, eye, ear, body cavities, bone, and from intravenous catheters which were not included in our series either). Routine cultures of skin or wounds had not been taken; therefore, the colonization rate of *S. marcescens* was not known to us.

The specimens had been routinely inoculated on blood agar, Desoxycholate agar, Chapman-Stone agar, Colymycin-Nalidixic acid(CNA)-blood agar, anaerobic Kanamycin-blood agar, and into fluid Thioglycollate Medium[1]. Identification of *S. marcescens* from desoxycholate agar proceeded according to methods described earlier (von Graevenitz and Fappiano). Antimicrobial sensitivity testing followed the Kirby-Bauer method (Bauer et al.).

Patient records were reviewed subsequently. All strains that were repeatedly isolated from the same patient showed identical sensitivities. Comparative statistical evaluation was done with the help of the fourfold contingency tests (Mainland and Murray).

Results and Discussion

Frequency

440 (0.4%) of *all* specimens received during the study period yielded *S. marcescens*. This frequency is twice that observed in 1964 to 1965 (Clayton and von Graevenitz); corresponding increases have been reported from other laboratories (Barrett et al.). Compared to such Enterobacteriaceae as *Escherichia coli*, *Klebsiella pneumoniae*, *Enterobacter cloacae*, *Enterobacter aerogenes*, and *Proteus mirabilis*, *S. marcescens* is still a rare bacterium to be isolated; and strains from soft tissue made up only 34 (7.8%) of all *S. marcescens* isolates (vs. 87% from urinary and respiratory tract sources). The actual incidence in soft tissue lesions is probably higher if one considers colonization as well.

Table 1 indicates that 85% of the strains isolated from soft tissue were found mixed with microorganisms commonly encountered in such infections, mostly in equal quantities. This percentage is significantly higher than the percentage of mixed *S. marcescens* cultures from other sources (Clayton and von Graevenitz). It equals that found in soft tissue infections with enterococci, anaerobic gram-negative rods, and indol-positive *Proteus* spp., but is much higher than that for similar infections with *E. coli*, *Enterobacter* spp., *Pseudomonas aeruginosa*, and *Staphylococcus aureus* (von Graevenitz, unpublished observations). The significance of this phenomenon is unknown but it may be related to a low virulence of *S. marcescens* (von Graevenitz, 1964).

However, the distribution of the concomitant organisms in our specimens is remarkably similar to their distribution in soft tissue infections in general. Enterococci were found in wounds on the trunk as well as on the extremities; their relatively high incidence is explained by the routine use of CNA blood agar which yields higher isolation rates for gram-positive cocci than blood agar (von Graevenitz et al., 1970).

Antimicrobial Sensitivity

Table 2 demonstrates that gentamicin was the only antibiotic effective against all strains, as has also been reported by others (Bodey et al., Wilfert et al., 1968, 1970). Except for a marked increase in resistance to kanamycin (38% resistant strains vs. none in 1966)—which goes along with an increased use of the drug (Wilfert et al., 1970), — sensitivity to other antimicrobials did not differ signifi-

---

[1] Source of media: BioQuest, Cockeysville, Md.

Table 1. *Occurrence of S. marcescens with other pathogens in cultures from soft tissues*[a]

Organisms	Occurrence in 100 cultures from soft tissues with growth %	Occurrence in 34 cultures from tissues with *S. marcescens* %
Enterococci	42	27.5
P. aeruginosa	34	17.7
S. aureus	28	27.5
E. coli	25	11.7
Klebsiella sp.	24	29.3
Proteus sp.	25	8.8
Beta-hemolytic streptococci	17	5.9
Enterobacter sp.	14	11.7
Candida sp.	11	8.8
Anaerobic gram-negative rods	10	2.9
Citrobacter/Levinea	8.5	5.9
Clostridium perfringens	8.5	0.0
Serratia marcescens	1.5	14.5[b]

[a] 88 % hospital-acquired and 12 % community-acquired strains, 85 % wounds and 15 % abscesses.

[b] *S. marscescens* in pure culture.

Table 2. *Antimicrobial sensitivities*

Fully sensitive to	Number of strains	%
Gentamicin	34	100
Nalidixic acid	27	79
Chloramphenicol[a]	25	73
Kanamycin	21	62
Streptomycin	16	47
Tetracycline	4	12
Nitrofurantoin	2	6
Two of these drugs	11	32
Three of these drugs	4	12
Four of these drugs	5	15
Five or more drugs	14	41

[a] See text.

cantly from that found in 1966 (VON GRAEVENITZ, 1967). Recent observations in our laboratory show that the percentage of *S. marcescens* strains resistant to several of the antimicrobials listed is now significantly higher in urinary tract isolates than in respiratory tract isolates—a feature not observed in 1966 but seen in strains of *Klebsiella* as well (EICKHOFF et al.). Isolates from blood and wound occupy a middle position. The percentage of chloramphenicol-sensitive strains may be misleading because M.I.C. values for this drug disagree with disc test results in *S. marcescens* (Bodey et al.; von Graevenitz, 1967). There was no correlation between sensitivity patterns and antibiotic therapy preceding the isolation of *S. marcescens*.

Sex and Age of Patients

During the observation period, there was an even age and sex distribution in hospital patients ranging from age 20 to 80. Sex distribution was also equal in our patients, but three-quarters of them were over 50 years old. Such age preference is typical for *S. marcescens* but also for nosocomial wound infections (Public Health Laboratory Service Report, 1960).

Site of Isolation and Origin of Strains

Table 3 shows that the most frequent sites of isolation were postoperative wounds on the abdomen and along the urinary tract and skin lesions on the legs

Table 3. *Sites of isolation*

Site	Number of strains		
	Postoperative wound	Skin lesion (cellulitis, laceration, necrosis)	Abscess
Head and neck	2	1	1
Arms	0	3	1
Chest	2	0	0
Abdomen	6	1	0
Urinary tract	6	0	2
Legs	2	6	0

(six patients each). In 16 patients, the same strain of *S. marcescens* was first isolated from sources other than the soft tissues (Table 4); the average time span between admission and isolation being 7 days—in contrast to 19 days in cases of primary isolation from the wound. Due to the absence of cultures from apparently "healthy" sites, the actual portal of entry for *S. marcescens* may have been missed in a few instances; we believe that in two cases of primary wound isolation the portal of entry was the urinary tract.

The final source was obviously a natural one (soil or water) in four (i.e., the community-acquired) cases, and IPPB machines that were used on the five patients with primary isolation from the respiratory tract. Such machines are common transmitters of respiratory infections with gram-negative rods in general, and *S. marcescens* in particular (Cabrera; Ringrose et al.; Sanders et al; Wilfert et al., 1970). Instrumentation had been performed on all eight patients in whom the urinary tract was the primary site of isolation; it is most frequently found in the history of patients with urinary tract infection due to *S. marcescens*.

The difference in the time span between admission and isolation quoted above could be explained by the larger inoculum and lower degree of local resistance that accompany respiratory and urinary tract infections.

Five of our cases obviously represented cross-infections, since strains of identical serotypes and antimicrobial sensitivities were found simultaneously in other patients on the same wards. Intermediary spread of *S. marcescens* through hands (SANDERS et al.), air (MAGNUSON and ELSTON), and irrigation solutions (CABRERA) has been suggested; we could find no identifiable source in the rest of our cases. Although the possibility of endogenous infection with *S. marcescens* through the gastrointestinal flora has been discounted (MAGNUSON and ELSTON) and stool or

Table 4. *Origin of strains*

S. marcescens first isolated from	Number of strains
Soft tissue	18
Urinary tract	8
Respiratory tract	5
Blood	1
Other sources	2

pharyngeal isolates have been rare (JOHANSON et al., CLAYTON and VON GRAEVE-NITZ, WILFERT et al., 1970), we would not dismiss it out of hand, since the isolation of *S. marcescens* from stool obviously requires highly selective media.

Preexisting Conditions

A very high percentage of patients with *S. marcescens* infection of the urinary or respiratory tract or of the blood have been found to suffer from an underlying disease (see reviews). Furthermore, the history of these patients often reveals previous hospitalizations, instrumentation, respiratory assistance, and anti-microbial treatment. As Table 5 demonstrates, these factors play a role in soft tissue infections with *S. marcescens* as well. 70% of our patients had undergone major surgery (lasting for more than 1 h) prior to the isolation, and 13 (38%) had drains inserted in the postoperative wounds. These factors are associated with a higher incidence of wound infection than is expected normally (Public Health Laboratory Service Report, 1960). In two cases, infection of arterial grafts occurred; such infections show a high incidence of gram-negative rods, particularly *S. marcescens* (CONN et al.).

Local Symptomatology

Since only obviously infected areas were cultured, the symptomatology did not differ from that observed in wound infections with gram-negative rods: redness, watery or purulent discharge, fluctuation where abscesses were present. Wounds with mixed and pure flora showed no differences in symptomatology. Fever attributable to the local process was present in 19 patients, two of them with *S. marcescens* in pure culture.

Hospital-Acquired and Community-Acquired Strains

Hospital-acquired *S. marcescens* strains were those that were not isolated from the patient at the time of admission or—in the absence of previous cultures—were cultured from "clean" areas; 23 of our strains unequivocally belonged in

Table 5. *Preexisting conditions*

Preexisting condition	Number of patients
Diseases	
Sequelae of hypertension and/or arteriosclerosis	11
Chronic urinary tract disease	9
Malignant tumor	8[a]
Local skin affection	7
Diabetes mellitus	7
Duodenal ulcer with bleeding and/or perforation	5
Obstructive jaundice	2
Alcoholism	2
Paralysis of lower extremities	2
Generalized skin disease	2
Endocarditis due to *Candida* sp.	1
Previous diagnostic or therapeutic measures	
Major surgery (over 1 h)	24
Hospitalization in past 12 months	19
Antimicrobial treatment prior to isolation of *S. marcescens*	23[b]
Urinary tract instrumentation	8
IPPB treatment	5
Steroid therapy	3
None	4[c]

[a] One case of leukemia.

[b] In seven cases, with drugs effective against *S. marcescens* in vitro.

[c] Community-acquired strains.

this category, 3 were probably hospital-acquired, and 4 were of indeterminate origin but caused, by definition, hospital-acquired infection (e.g., from cholecystectomy wounds). Twenty-two patients with clearly or probably hospital-acquired strains were on surgical or urological wards.

Four strains were community-acquired. Similar to two such strains reported earlier (von Graevenitz, 1964), they were isolated from varicose ulcers or from ischemic lesions from diabetic patients. The patients' average age was 75 years (vs. 61 in the hospital-acquired group), they had not been previously treated with antimicrobials (as had 78% of the hospital-acquired group), and had localized infections with multiple bacteria that improved on therapy which was not specifically directed against *S. marcescens*. All community-acquired strains were sensitive to at least five of the antimicrobials listed in Table 2. Noteworthy is the obvious community origin of the strains of *S. marcescens* that occurred together with an anaerobe in the first infection (colonization ?) with *S. marcescens* reported in the literature (DU BOIS ST.-SÉVRIN).

Postoperative Wound Infections Yielding *S. marcescens*

Twenty postoperative wounds (58% of all soft tissue cultures with *S. marcescens*) yielded the organism; 18 of them are the ones listed in Table 3, and in 2, superinfection of a draining abscess had occurred. Only five (25%) were considered "clean". *Preoperative* cultures from sites other than the wound had only been positive for *S. marcescens* in 2 patients; in 10 (50%), *S. marcescens* had appeared *post*operatively at other sites and had then spread to the wound. The average time span between operation and first isolation of *S. marcescens* from the wound was 9.6 days. In this regard, *S. marcescens* resembles coliform bacteria which tend to appear in the second week in wound infections (BARBER), in contrast to staphylococci in the first and *Ps. aeruginosa* in the third week. The incidence of previous antimicrobial treatment was not significantly higher in the postoperative wound infection group than in the rest of the cases.

Contribution of *S. marcescens* to Disease

In order to assess the contribution of *S. marcescens* to the disease process, a combined evaluation of previous culture results, the quantity of S. *marcescens* in relation to other bacteria present, and the effect of specific antimicrobial treatment against *S. marcescens* (as shown in follow-up cultures) was undertaken.

Table 6 shows the effect of various treatment regimens. Remarkable is the recovery, in spite of inappropriate treatment, of eight patients in whom *S. marcescens* had been present locally only—suggesting a saprophytic existence of *S. marcescens*. On the other hand, seven patients with "systemic" findings of *S. marcescens* (i.e., on several sites) did not improve despite appropriate chemotherapy. This was probably due to a malfunction of the normal defense mechanisms which were influenced by the underlying disease(s) and on which the effect of antimicrobial treatment depends in part (WEINSTEIN and DALTON). A high failure rate of anti-*S. marcescens* chemotherapy in cancer patients has been reported recently (BODEY et al.).

It can be seen from Table 7 that the "indeterminate" category is rather large, due to the frequent occurrence of *S. marcescens* with other potential pathogens. While superinfection with *S. marcescens* was observed in six patients, its contributory effect could not be accurately evaluated. However, it can be stated that in the majority of cases with purely local disease, *S. marcescens* must have existed as a saprophyte. When "systemic" presence of *S. marcescens* was observed, saprophytic existence was infrequent, and the contributory effect extended to the local as well as to the "systemic" process.

Ten patients died, all with hospital-acquired strains. In five, *S. marcescens* contributed to the fatal outcome, and always in the form of a "systemic" infection (including three cases of S. marcescens septicemia). Localized infections were not lethal. Distribution of the previously discussed factors (sex, age, sensitivities, etc.) did not differ in this group from the rest.

Table 6. *Effect of antimicrobial treatment for S. marcescens*

Treatment with Antimicrobials	Clinical effect	Local infection present only	Local and "systemic" infection present
Effective[a] in vitro	improved	3	3
	not improved	0	7
Ineffective[b] in vitro	improved	8	0
	not improved	0	3
None or non-specific	improved	5	2
	not improved	0	1

[a] Effective against *S. marcescens*.
[b] Ineffective against *S. marcescens* but effective against other bacteria present.

Table 7. *Contribution of S. marcescens to disease*

Effect	Local infection present only	Local and "systemic" infection present	Total
Contributory	3	10	13
Most likely non-contributory	8	3	11
Indeterminate	7	3	10

Description of an Unusual Case

A 68 year old diabetic woman was transferred to us from an outside hospital where she had been treated with oral steroids for an exfoliative dermatitis which had developed after phenylbutazone intake. On admission, she presented with multiple denuded skin areas on head, trunk, and extremities, some of them obviously infected. A culture of urine taken on admission grew *S. marcescens* and *Klebsiella pneumoniae* (both more than 100,000/ml); and cultures from several infected sites yielded *S. marcescens* as well. Both isolates of *S. marcescens* were sensitive to gentamicin, nalidixic acid, kanamycin, chloramphenicol, streptomycin, and tetracycline. The patient developed septicemia with *S. marcescens* 2 days after admission and was treated with tetracycline. This regimen led to the disappearance of *S. marcescens* from the blood and urine, but the urinary tract became superinfected with *Proteus mirabilis*, and cultures of the skin lesions now grew, in addition to *S. marcescens, Ps. aeruginosa, P. mirabilis*, and yeasts. The patient improved on intensive treatment with kanamycin. However, 18 days after admission she lapsed into a coma and developed hemiparesis. She died 3 days later; a tentative diagnosis of a space-occupying lesion had been made. Autopsy revealed multiple brain abscesses from which *S. marcescens* was cultured.

This case illustrates some of the features of soft tissue infection with *S. marcescens* that we have outlined.

Summary

Serratia marcescens has been isolated with increasing frequency in the past few years, but only 34 (7.8%) of all strains isolated in a 22-month period came from soft tissue infections. Such strains were more sensitive to antimicrobials than urinary tract isolates. More than one-half came from abdominal and urological wounds and from leg lesions. Possible sources include other sites on the patient colonized or infected with *S. marcescens*, patients on the same ward, inanimate vectors (e.g., respiratory equipment), soil, and water. There was a significant time difference between (early) isolation of *S. marcescens* from other sites and (late) isolation from soft tissue infections after admission. Underlying disease which weakened local or general defense mechanisms and previous therapeutic measures (instrumentation, antimicrobial treatment, etc.) were found in the history of a high percentage of our patients. 88% acquired the infection in the hospital; superinfection was noted in 6%. In postoperative wounds, *S. marcescens* appeared in the second week. A definite contribution to the disease process could be established in 13 instances only; this effect was more often associated with "systemic" disease due to *S. marcescens*, while in purely localized infections, *S. marcescens* tended to exist as a saprophyte.

References

BARBER, M.: Wound healing. Lister Centenary Symposium, Glasgow. London: Churchill 1966.

BARRETT, F. F., CASEY, J. I., FINLAND, M.: Infections and antibiotic usage among patients at Boston City Hospital, February 1967. New Engl. J. Med. **278**, 5—9 (1968).

BAUER, A. W., KIRBY, W. M. M., SHERRIS, J. C., TURCK, M.: Antibiotic susceptibility testing by a standardized single disk method. Amer. J. clin. Path. **45**, 493—496 (1966).

BODEY, G. P., RODRIGUEZ, V., SMITH, J. P.: *Serratia sp.* infections in cancer patients. Cancer (Philad.) **25**, 199—205 (1970).

CABRERA, H. A.: An outbreak of *Serratia marcescens* and its control. Arch. intern. Med. **123**, 650—655 (1969).

CLAYTON, E., VON GRAEVENITZ, A.: Nonpigmented *Serratia marcescens*. J. Amer. med. Ass. **197**, 1059—1064 (1966).

CONN, J. H., HARDY, J. D., CHAVEZ, C. M., FAIN, W. R.: Infected arterial grafts: Experience in 22 cases with emphasis on unusual bacteria and technics. Ann. Surg. **171**, 704—713 (1970).

DU BOIS ST.-SÉVRIN: Panaris de pêcheurs et microbes rouges de la sardine. Ann. Inst. Pasteur 8, 152—160 (1894).

EICKHOFF, T. C., STEINHAUER, B. W., FINLAND, M.: The *Klebsiella-Enterobacter-Serratia* division. Biochemical and serologic characteristics and susceptibility to antibiotics. Ann. intern. Med. **65**, 1163—1179 (1966).

EWING, W. H., JOHNSON, J. G., DAVIES, B. R.: The occurrence of *Serratia marcescens* in nosocomial infections. Atlanta, Ga.: Communicable Disease Center 1962.

FIELDS, B. N., UWAYDAH, M. M., KUNZ, L. J., SWARTZ, M. N.: The so-called "Paracolon" bacteria. A bacteriologic and clinical reappraisal. Amer. J. Med. **42**, 89—106 (1967).

GALE, D., SONNENWIRTH, A. C.: Frequent human isolation of *Serratia marcescens*. Arch. intern. Med. **109**, 414—421 (1962).

JOHANSON, W. G., PIERCE, A. K., SANFORD, J. P.: Changing pharyngeal bacterial flora of hospitalized patients. Emergence of gram-negative bacilli. New Engl. J. Med. **281**, 1137 to 1140 (1969).

MAGNUSON, C. W., ELSTON, H. R.: Infections by nonpigmented *Serratia*. Report of seven cases. Ann. intern. Med. **65**, 409—418 (1966).

MAINLAND, D., MURRAY, I. M.: Tables for use in four-fold contingency tests. Science **116**, 591—594 (1952).

PUBLIC HEALTH LABORATORY SERVICE. Report. Incidence of surgical wound infection in England and Wales. Lancet **1960 II**, 659—663.

RINGROSE, R. E., McKOWN, B., FELTON, F. G., BARCLAY, B. O., MUCHMORE, H. G., RHOADES, E. R.: A hospital outbreak of *Serratia marcescens* associated with ultrasonic nebulizers. Ann. intern. Med. **69**, 719—729 (1968).

SANDERS, C. V., LUBY, J. P., JOHANSON, W. G., BARNETT, J. A., SANFORD, J. P.: *Serratia marcescens* infection from inhalation therapy medications: nosocomial outbreak. Ann. intern. Med. **73**, 15—21 (1970).

VON GRAEVENITZ, A.: Über *Serratia*-Infektionen beim Menschen. Path. et Microbiol. (Basel) **27**, 235—247 (1964).

— Sensitivity studies on *Serratia* strains from clinical specimens. Chemotherapia (Basel) **12**, 215—225 (1967).

— FAPPIANO, A.: Schnelle und ökonomische Identifizierung gramnegativer Stäbchen von Desoxycholat-Agar. Zbl. Bakt., I. Abt. Orig. **212**, 500—505 (1970).

— STROUSE, A., GRINSTEAD, C.: Bacteria that can be isolated and aren't. Amer. J. Med. Techn. **36**, 565—573 (1970).

WEINSTEIN, L., DALTON, A. C.: Host determinants of response to antimicrobial agents (concl.). New Engl. J. Med. **279**, 580—588 (1968).

WILFERT, J. N., BARRETT, F. F., KASS, E. H.: Bacteremia due to *Serratia marcescens*. New Engl. J. Med. **279**, 286—289 (1968).

— — EWING, W. H., FINLAND, M., KASS, E. H.: *Serratia marcescens*: Biochemical, serological, and epidemiological characteristics and antibiotic susceptibility of strains isolated at Boston City Hospital. Appl. Microbiol. **19**, 345—352 (1970).

Prof. Dr. A. VON GRAEVENITZ
c/o Yale-New Haven Hospital
789 Howard Avenue
New Haven, Connecticut 06504 (U.S.A.)

Discussion

WYSOCKI: Prof. VON GRAEVENITZ, we have not yet seen any soft tissue infection caused by Serratia in our patients. Perhaps our laboratory failed to detect these organisms, but we have recently seen two cases of meningitis following neurosurgical operations. I should like to ask you how often have you seen meningitis caused by Serratia—what is your antimicrobial therapy in these infections?

VON GRAEVENITZ: I can only remember one case. We became aware of Serratia only in 1963 after the report of a fairly extensive survey of Serratia from the Communicable Disease Center had appeared. Treatment does depend upon the antimicrobial sensitivity of the organisms. If you suspect this organism to be present but do not have the results of sensitivity tests at the time, the most reliable drug right now would be gentamicin, followed by kanamycin, and maybe chloramphenicol.

I should be careful to point out that the other authors and we, ourselves, have shown that MIC's with chloramphenicol correlate rather poorly with disc sensitivity results in Serratia. Quite often the organism is diagnosed as "Paracolon", whatever that is.

GOULD: May I ask Prof. VON GRAEVENITZ what his experience has been with Serratia and closely allied organisms in relation to antiseptics in his unit ? We have found that these organisms are particularly resistant to chlorhexadine and this has been responsible for the spread of this organism to some soft tissue during dressings and probing of wound and, in two instances, it was followed by meningitis of the type described by Dr. WYSOCKI. Do you know of any other particularly ineffective antiseptic substances against these strains ? Have you any experience with this ?

VON GRAEVENITZ: Not that I could document! I do have the feeling that the quarternary ammonium compounds are not particularly effective against Serratia but that glutaraldehyde (in the form of Cidex) is quite effective. For the specific disinfection of inhalation therapy equipment, it is recommended that 0.2% acetic acid be used. In order to minimise the risk of transmission. We have also asked the inhalation therapy department to use one machine on one patient at one time only.

PULVERER: We have a set of cultures of Serratia. May I ask you to send us strains so that we can prove if our cultures are good for phage typing.

VON GRAEVENITZ: I would be happy to do so.

KASS: I just want to re-emphasize this frequency which seems to show up in a hospital. We isolate from 30 to 50 strains a day from all sources.

PULVERER: May I ask what does it mean in percentage of your isolates ?

KASS: A few percent among several hundred cultures a day.

Bayer-Symposium III, 145—154 (1971)
© by Springer-Verlag 1971

Septic Infections by Bacteria of Low Pathogenicity in Patients with Resistance Reduced by Chemotherapy

O. R. Gsell

With 1 Figure

The increasing incidence of septic infections by bacteria of low pathogenicity is clinically remarkable in two respects. The clinician wonders why opportunistic microbes, mainly gram-negative bacteria, otherwise known as harmless, have now become the cause of severe disease. On the one hand, there is no reason to suppose an increase in the pathogenicity of these bacteria. They do not form

Table 1. *Causes of the increasing incidence of septic infections by gram-negative organisms*

1. Use of antibiotics and sulfonamides to which resistance has developed.
2. Increasing incidence of pancytopenia as a side-effect of therapy
3. The advent of cytostatics and immunosuppressives.
4. Increasing application of surgical instrumentation measures.

a well-defined group, but they differ a great deal; strains of micro-organisms that are in no way related, are also found as pathogens of the same severe infections.

On the other hand, the usual reasons for a reduction of host resistance on the part of the human body are unlikely to be a cause. There have been reductions of resistance at all times. The effects of poor hygienic conditions, of malnutrition, of war, and especially the circumstances of the high infant mortality in the third world do not apply to our problem today. Such damages have always induced an increase in the incidence of infections, but those infections were due to the long known pathogens. The individual bodily damages encountered in civilized areas, — for example alcoholism, drug abuse, and increase of constitutional diseases, such as diabetes, and eventually overaging, with more arteriosclerosis and cancer, are recognized causes of increasing morbidity and mortality but not of the infections by bacteria of low pathogenicity here under discussion.

We have to consider *damages which until recently did not occur* as the basis of the new phenomenon (see Table 1).

One cause has been experimentally and clinically clarified—the *world wide use of antibiotics* during which part of the pathogenic cocci, in particular gram-positive cocci, are eliminated and, as a secondary phenomen, gram-negative organisms become predominant and may become pathogenic. In particular infections, of the urinary, respiratory and intestinal organs show an increased preponderance of gram-negative bacteria. This process has been enhanced by *hospitalism* in the form of micro-organisms resistant to sulfonamides and antibiotics, promoted by the use of these therapeutics. Among the clinical publications, those by M. FINLAND should be pointed out. As early as about the close of the 1950's he provided statistical foundations concerning the frequency of gram-negative bacteremias.

The second cause is rooted in a *side-effect of the antibiotics*. They can damage an organ that has an essential function in the defense against infection—the bone

Table 2. *Bacteremia due to bacteria of low pathogenicity*

Sex	Age	Microorganisms-sepsis	Chemotherapy	Basic disease	Result
F	72	*Bac. subtilis*	Cytostatics: a) Onkovin b) Fluouracil c) Methotrexate d) Prednisone	Metast. Mamma Ca with sec. pancytopenia	Cured
F	58	a) Spirilla b) Staphylococci c) Cytomegaly	a) Leukeran b) Neomercazol c) Prednisone	Chron. Lymphadenosis + Hyperthyrosis + Diabetes mellitus	Cured
M	52	Pseudomonas aerogenes	a) Endoxan b) Prednisone	Chron. lymphatic Leukemia	+
M	80	*E. coli* — Fungal pneumonia	a) Vincristin b) Prednisone	Chron. lymphosarcomatosis with sec. pancytopenia	+
M	49	Paracoli	Imurel 1,400 mg	Liver cirrhosis and chron. alcoholism	+
M	49	a) Proteus b) Mimea c) *E. cloacae*	Imurel 400 mg	Subacute hepatitis + rheumatoid arthritis	Cured
F	47	Staphylococci	Imurel 4,700 mg + Methatrexate 100 mg + Prednisone	Lupus erythematosis with sec. pancytopenia	+

marrow. This has led to an increased incidence of pancytopenia, and particularly agranulocytosis, which favour the development of septic diseases due to the usual pathogenic bacteria, as well as the now more frequent bacteria of low pathogenicity.

The third cause is the intensive administration of *cytotoxic chemotherapeutics* which have only become available during the past 10 years. Especially in this connection, diseases are caused by opportunistic organisms which are already present in the body as saprophytes and are enhanced by the reduction of resistance caused by the diseases requiring the use of such chemotherapeutics. Therapy with *cytostatic agents* in cancer and with *immunosuppressive therapy* have led to septic infections by bacteria of low pathogenicity which formerly were not observed.

Seven recently observed examples from our own experience may serve as illustrations (see Table 2).

Case 1

M. M. is a 72 year-old woman, who at the age of 68 in 1966 had an operation for *mammary carcinoma* and post-operative irradiation. One year later skin metastases appeared and, after 2 years, bone metastases. She made a good recovery with X-ray therapy plus administration of prednisone and "Decadurabolin". For half a year she went without treatment. Then in November 1969 she had a spontaneous fracture of a thoracic vertebra due to metastases. After admission on November 18, 1969 she received *quadruple cytostatic* chemotherapy until January 22, 1970: Oncovin, 5 mg, fluorouracil 1,500 mg, methotrexate 13.5 mg, total doses, and prednisone 30 mg daily. On January 23, 1970 panmyelopathy was detected and cytostatic treatment withdrawn. W.B.C. 1,900 (neutrophils about 60 %) anemia (Hb 8.1 g- %, erythrocytes 2.24 million), thrombo-cytopenia (22,000 platelets). She developed fever and symptoms of influenza for 4 days, and thereafter had septic temperatures. Blood cultures on January 27 was negative, but on February 2 a culture yielded a pure growth of *Bac. subtilis* (Prof. REBER). Gentamicin 120 mg daily was given for 9 days and the patient became completely afebrile within 10 days. The W.B.C. February 6, 1970 was up to 7,240; platelet count on February 19 was 551,000. From the middle of February on, the patient made a pleasant recovery. The patient was restored to the previous stage and later on showed slow progression of metastases and she died July 1970.

Summary: In a patient with generalized metastases of a mammary carcinoma, mainly with bone involvement, quadruple cytostatic chemotherapy resulted in an acute toxic panmyelopathy after 2 months. The chemotherapy was discontinued, but a septic condition developed on the 10th day, and the blood culture grew *Bac. subtilis*. The sepsis was controlled with gentamicin treatment, the malignant condition was not changed but the pancytopenia disappeared in 2 weeks.

Case 2

G. O., a 58 year-old woman had diabetes mellitus for 10 years, controlled with 50 units of insulin daily. In December 1969 a diagnosis of a *toxic adenoma of the thyroid* (PBI 19.6 γ- %) and *chronic lymphadenosis* with lymph-node swelling was made. The W.B.C. was about 15,000, lymphocytes 85 %, Hb 8.2 %, erythrocytes 2.6 million. From January 26 until the end of February she received treatment with Leukeran 4 mg daily. On March 12, 1970 a therapeutic dose of radioactive iodine was given. She was admitted to the hospital March 13 with Hb 5.9 g- %. Blood transfusions provoked intolerance reactions. On March 13 administration of prednisone, 100 mg daily, was started and given until April 6, then the dose was reduced to 10 mg daily until March 26. From March 16 until April 4, 1970 she received Neomercazol, 100 mg daily. On March 25, 1970 she became febrile and had thrombophlebitis of the left lower leg with persistent fever. In the middle of April the fever was septic in type. On April 20, 1970 the W.B.C. was 4,100, neutrophils 82 %, lymphocytes 15 %, Hb 9.3. Blood culture gave a pure growth of *Spirillium* identified by Prof. LÖFFLER as *Spirillium ehrenberg*, with typical flagellae seen by electronmicroscopy (see Fig. 1). She became afebrile on treatment with cloxacillin, 14 g in 8 days. After 3 weeks she had a second septic episode, with blood cultures twice positive for *Staphylococcus aureus*, this was controlled with oxacillin 2 g daily for 10 days. She again made a good recovery and became afebrile. During the following months her general well-being was stationary with chronic lymphadenosis. It should be mentioned that the immunofluorescence titre for cytomegalovirus antibody (Dr. KRECH) showed a remarkable rise: from 1:60 on April 23 to 1:160, on April 29 and May 28.

Summary: A 58 year-old woman with compensated diabetes received cytostatic therapy with Neuomercazol and prednisone for chronic lymphadenosis and hyperthyrotoxicosis. The first septic episode yielded *Spirillium* in the blood culture, the second *Staphylococcus*. Both were controlled by antibiotic treatment and the previous condition restored. Serological tests showed simultaneous activation of a cytomegalcovirus infection.

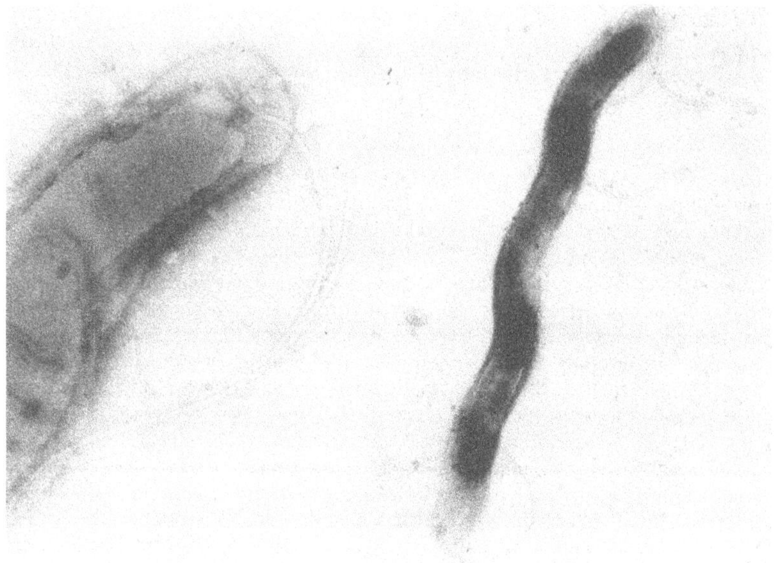

Fig. 1. *Spirillium ehrenberg* (electron microscopy 35,000 ×, Inst. of Microbiology, Basel), case 2

Case 3

St. A., was a 52 year-old man in whom a diagnosis of chronic lymphadenosis was made in 1966, when he was given gland irradiation. From 1967 to 1969 he had no treatment and no change in his general well-being. On April 10, 1970 he complained of tiredness and an increase of glandular swellings. On May 11, 1970 his W.B.C. was 66,000, lymphocytes 91 %, Hb 6.0 %, erythrocytes 1.5 million and platelets 67,000. On May 14 he was started on treatment with *Endoxan*, 50 mg daily (only 700 mg total) and prednisone, 50 mg daily until May 29. On May 26 he began to have fever and on May 29 he was admitted to the hospital where a diagnosis of *pseudomonas sepsis* was made (anemia, Hb 4.89 %, erythrocytes 1,4 million, W.B.C. 38,200, lymphocytes 92 %, thrombocytes 46,000) and treatment with gentamicin and ampicillin were ineffective and the patient died on June 8, 1970. Autopsy revealed pseudomonas meningitis and sepsis, in addition to leukemic involvement of lymph nodes, spleen and liver and displacement of the blood forming bone marrow.

Summary: Fatal *pseudomonas sepsis* occurred after 14 days treatment with Endoxan and prednisone in a case of chronic lymphatic leukemia.

Case 4

W. A., a 80 year-old man with *chronic lymphosarcomatosis* and extensive glandular involvement but no enlargement of spleen or liver, received irradiation treatment for $1^1/_4$ years. Beginning July 14 he was given prednisone 100 mg, then 50 mg daily for a total of 1,500 mg in 2/1 days, and *Vincristin* for a total of 4 g. in 3 weeks. After August 19 he developed fever, *pancytopenia* with agranulocytosis and purpura. The W.B.C. on August 24 was 1,500 with 98 % lymphocytes, 1 % neutrophils, 1 % monocytes, Hb 7.8 g- %, platelets 20,000. Blood cultures yielded *E. coli*. The patient died on August 26. Autopsy showed: Coli sepsis, leukemic lymphadenosis, pneumonia with abscess, and fungal infection in the lung.

Summary: Escherichia coli sepsis occurred after 3 weeks of treatment with Vincristin and prednisone in the course of which pancytopenia developed in a 80 year-old man with chronic lymphadenosis. The patient died from sepsis and fungal pneumonia.

Case 5

M. R., a 49 year-old man with a history of *rheumatoid arthritis* for 12 years was admitted on October 2, 1969 with *hepatitis*, probably inoculation hepatitis. At no time had he received corticosteroids. A diagnosis of active *chronic progressive hepatitis* was established by liver biopsy, serum bilirubin was 13 mg- %, SGOT 33, SGPT 20 i.u., 33 B units alkaline phosphatase. On October 18, W.B.C. was 10,000, 46 % stab cells 38 segmented cells, eos 3 %, mono 7 %, lymphocytes 6 %, Hb 11.5 g- %, platelet count 160,000. He was started on Imurel 100 mg daily. After 3 days he became febrile as of the 4th day, had high febrile and a septic state with a pustular exanthema, bronchopneumonia and peritoneal irritation. Blood culture on October 19 was positive, yielding *Bac. proteus, Mima polymorpha, Enterobacter cloacae* (Prof. REBER). On October 20 only Proteus was grown from the blood culture. Therapy with penicillin, streptomycin fluid infusions, then gentamicin checked the dangerous conditions. On October 24, W.B.C. was 16,000 and thereafter there was no fever. Hepatitis persisted but slowly improved within 3 months.

Summary: Development of sepsis, presenting a polymicrobial bacteremia with a mixed flora which comprised gram-negative organisms, Proteus, *Mima polymorpha, E. cloacae* after 4 days' administration of *Imurel* (400 mg) for active aggressive hepatitis. The infection was cured with antibiotic therapy.

Case 6

M. F., a 49 year-old teacher, a chronic alcoholic, had chronic active *cirrhosis of the liver* for 5 years and in addition, *thrombocytopenia* with platelet values of 30,000 to 40,000 for 3 years. In July 1968, the hemorrhagic diathesis became worse despite cortisone treatment, and on August 2, 1968 Imurel 3 mg, t.d.s. was started. A fortnight later on August 16, after a total of 1,100 mg Imurel, ascites and a rapidly progressing fever with septic condition and peritonitis occurred. A diagnosis of intestinal perforation with peritonitis was made. Blood culture grew *Paracolon bacillus* (GSELL), W.B.C. was 10,800, platelets 17,000, Hb 14.8g- %. On August 24 despite antibiotic therapy the patient died in shock.

Summary: In a case of long standing cirrhosis of the liver and thrombocytopenia in a chronic alcoholic, sepsis with *Paracolon bacillus* occurred after 14 days of Imurel treatment. Three days later the patient died of peritonitis and shock resulting from perforation of the bowel.

Case 7

P. M., a 47 year-old woman had *lupus erythematosus* with remissions and relapses for 14 years. On June 5, 1967 because of a reactivation of the disease, *Imurel* 50 mg twice daily was started. Because of persistent limb pains, the treatment was stopped after a total dose of 2.9 g on July 2. No improvement had been achieved. From July 3 onwards the patient received *methotrexate*, 2,5 mg daily, which after an interruption between July 10 and 18, because of purpura and exanthema, was continued to a total of 70 mg, until August 9. Prednisone was administered from January 31, until September 19, in 30 mg daily dosage. No improvement occurred, and therefore a *second course* of *Imurel* was given from August 10, initially 100 mg daily, from August 18, 200 mg, from August 22, 250 mg. After 4.7 g the drug was stopped on September 2 when the W.B.C. was 2,700 and with 69 % neutrophils, Hb 12.4 %. Methotrexate 2,5 mg daily was given from September 2 to 13. From September 6 she had *staphylococcal sepsis* with high fever and bronchopneumonia with masses of staphylococci in the sputum. With the septic infection there was a *pancytopenia*. On August 13 the W.B.C. was 1,300, and on the next day 700; the Hb 6.9 % and platelets 3,500 and on August 14 the patient died.

Summary: Pancytopenia developed in a patient with long standing lupus erythematosus after 23 days of treatment with Imurel 4.7 g and intermittent methotrexate and was followed by *staphylococcal sepsis* which terminated fatally within 9 days.

The pathogens causing the sepsis in these seven cases were very different microorganisms, for example, gram-negative bacteria such as *E. coli*, Paracolon-

Enterobacteriaceae, *Mima polymorpha (B. antitratum)*, Proteus, *Pseudomonas aeruginosa* and as rarities, *B. subtilis* and *Spirillum ehrenberg* and in one case *Staphylococcus aureus. The basic conditions* were malignant blood diseases, carcinoma, subacute liver disease, lupus erythematosus, diabetes mellitus and hyperthyroidism. In more than half the cases the bacteremia was preceded by pancytopenia resulting from the chemotherapy given for the basic disease.

The *direct cause* for the sepsis in four cases was *cytostatic chemotherapy*, always combined with prednisone, and in three cases *immunosuppressive therapy* with Imurel in varying high dosage alone or combined with Neomercazol, or methotrexate, and, in one case, only prednisone. It is well known that cytostatics lead to pancytopenia and in their present form must do so to become fully effective. The necessary high dosage of these chemotherapeutics and the frequent combination of several drugs

Table 3. *Factors possibly predisposing to bacteremia, 113 cases 1955—1959 (*McHENRY *et al., 1962)*

	%
Malignant disease	17
Hematologic disease	13
Diabetes mellitus	11
Severe hepatic disease	5
Antibiotic induced alterations of normal flora	19
Adrenal cortical steroids	14
Toxin chemotherapeutic agents	5

are responsible for the increasing number of cases of secondary gram-negative bacteremia as a result of this treatment. Pancytopenia is also a threat with immunosuppressive therapy, the indication for which must therefore by considered very seriously, since the basic diseases for which it is considered are not by themselves malignant, for example, liver disease (DANIELI et al.), rheumatoid arthritis (see DEICHER et al.) lupus erythematosus. Sepsis can develop without pancytopenia (as in case 5).

The *occurrence* of septic diseases due to opportunistic, often gram-negative microorganisms, is new in several respects, for example:

1. As a *result of modern chemotherapy* damaging cells or the cellular membrane, especially the cells of the bone marrow, and permitting the body's own flora to assume pathogenic action.

2. As a result of *advances in surgical instrumentation* for example, tracheal canulas, intubation, venous and arterial catheters, urological instrumentation, grafting of plastics, which are usually associated with antibiotic therapy and favour the invasion of pathogenic organisms into the blood stream. The statistical results of McHENRY et al. (1962) concerning the gram-negative bacteremias observed in the Mayo Clinic till 1959 are shown in Table 3. The authors noted toxic chemotherapeutics as agents which predisposed to diminution of the host's resistance

in only 5%. Since then the situation has entirely changed so that an exact analysis now reveals this effect often in more than 50% of cases.

3. *As a result of advances in laboratory technique* microorganisms can be cultured and isolated which in the past received little attention in human pathology. The different names used in microbiology produce difficulties. Most of the techniques are still reserved for specialized laboratories. With the gram-negative bacteria have been classified, besides *Enterobacteriaceae* according to the classification of EWING and EDWARDS (see Table 4), the *non-fermentative organisms* which do not ferment carbohydrates. These comprise *Bordetella bronchiseptica*, *Alcaligenes* species, the *Pseudomonas group*, *Mimea-Herellea* group and *Flavobacteria*.

GARDNER *et al.* found among 1,505 gram-negative bacteria isolated from blood, sputum, urine and wounds in a large hospital the following frequency (see Table 5). Owing to modern laboratory techniques more and more different microorganisms which produce bacteremia, for example *Bacillus subtilis*, Corynebacterium, Clostridium, Spirillium, are found.

Table 4. *Enterobacteriaceae (classification of* EWING *and* EDWARDS*)*

1. Shigella—Escherichia
2. Salmonella—Arizona—Citrobacter—Edwardsiella
3. Klebsiella—Aerobacter—Hafnia—Serratia
4. Proteus—Providencia

Particularly *unfavourable* is the *occurrence of multiple pathogens* in septicemias. HOCHSTEIN et al. distinguishes two groups, one in which more than one microorganism is found by blood culture (in 7.8% of their sepsis patients) and the second group (10%) in which the pathogen grown in the initial blood culture is replaced within 30 days by another one (change of microrganisme) as for example, in case 5. BODEY et al. observed among 420 bacteremias in acute leukemia, 54 cases with multiple organisms. They made on average six blood cultures per patient. Of these 54 cases, 50 were fatal. Most of the patients had marked leukopenia at the onset of the sepsis. In 59% of the cases, gram-negative organisms were found as the first intruders. Unfavourable prognosis does not apply to our two cases with multiple pathogens. *Polymicrobial bacteremia*, with isolation of two or more microganisms from the same blood sample, was confirmed in 46 patients, that is, 6% of all patients with bacteriologically established bacteremia seen by HERMANS and WASHINGTON. The mortality was 37%. A relatively benign clostridial bacteremia was found in four patients. The rare entity of polymicrobial endocarditis can easily be overlooked; it was seen in three patients.

The prognosis is grave in gram-negative *sepsis with endotoxic shock*, for which BLAIR et al. reported a 70 to 75% mortality rate. Shock was present in 38% of the gram-negative bacteremias.

In Switzerland, OECHSLIN et al. reported, as early as 1962, six cases of sepsis due to gram-negative bacteria associated with dangerous toxic shock, five of which terminated fatally. E. BECK described a case of proteus sepsis with shock and empyema. W.MEYER (1966) reported successful treatment consisting of replenishment of the circulatory volume with dextran and the administration of anti-adrenergic substances and corticosteroids in high doses. Of the 37 patients with gram-negative toxic shock reported by ENDERLIN et al. (1967), two-thirds had mixed infections, in one-third, one pathogen was detected, in 30 the condition

Table 5. *Relative frequency of gram-negative bacilli in clinical specimens (June 1967)* (GARDNER *et al.*)

Organism	Specimen					
	Urine	Sputum	Wound	Blood	Other	Totals
Nonfermentative species						
Bordetella bronchiseptica	0	2	—	—	—	2
Alcaligenes species	—	—	—	—	—	0
Pseudomonas maltophilia	4	8	2	—	—	14
Pseudomonas species (others)	4	2	3	—	—	9
Mima polymorpha	4	2	—	—	—	6
Herellea vaginicola	11	12	11	1	—	35
Pseudomonas aeruginosa	100	107	59	2	—	268
Flavobacteria	—	2	—	—	—	2
Enterobacteriaceae						
Escherichia coli	313	41	65	6	2	427
Klebsiella pneumoniae	203	109	53	15	2	387
Enterobacter	32	31	21	8	—	92
Proteus						
mirabilis	97	7	10	2	1	117
rettgeri	3	—	1	—	—	4
morganii	24	2	14	—	—	40
vulgaris	1	1	2	—	—	4
Serratia marcescens	57	5	—	1	—	63
Citrobacter freundii	7	6	2	—	—	15
Providencia	18	—	—	—	—	18
Hafnia	—	2	—	—	—	2
Totals	878	339	248	35	5	1,505

developed after abdominal surgery, and in three quarters it was combined with peritonitis following intestinal perforation or leakage at the suture line.

ALTEMEIER reviewed 398 cases (1955 to 1967) and found *E. coli* in 35%, *Klebsiella-Aerobacter* in 22%, *Pseudomonas aeruginosa* in 14%, Proteus 13%. Urogenital infections predominated and respiratory infections ranked second.

As concerns the *host's condition*, the basic disease is important for the prognosis. FREID and VOSTI distinguished three groups among their 270 bacteremias in which there was 36% mortality rate:

1. Rapidly progressive disease—for example, acute leukemias and other diseases rapidly leading to death, in which case only 14% survived the bacteremia.

2. Ultimately fatal disease—for example, metastatic malignancies, chronic leukemias, lymphomas, chronic uremia, immunological disease with renal involvement in which 54% survived the bacteremia.

3. Non-fatal basic diseases with a 84% survival (see Table 6).

In non-fatal diseases, immunosuppressives and corticosteroids are less often used than in the fatal disease groups. The more favourable prognosis of gram-negative bacteremia in non-fatal basic disease seems to depend on early antibiotic therapy (see McCABE and JACKSON).

It is no longer permissable to limit the therapy of septic infections, especially in pancytopenia, and toxic cases (W.B.C. under 1,000) to immediately beginning antibiotic treatment, mainly with tetracycline and the more recent

Table 6. *Fatality ratios according to severity of underlying disease*
(FREID *and* VOSTI, *1970*)

	%
Rapidly fatal	90
Ultimately fatal	84
Non fatal	14
Total	36

derivatives, but replenishment of fluid, electrolyte balance, correction of hypovolemia are equally important. Practically most patients need therapy in an intensive care unit and often require strict isolation.

Summary

The increasing importance of septic infections due to microorganisms of low pathogenicity in patients receiving chemotherapy and immunosuppressive treatment is demonstrated on the basis of cases from personal experience. Not only gram-negative bacteremias due to *Enterobacteriacae* and the group of non-fermentative organisms were observed, but in the own cases *Bacillus subtilis* and Spirillium also grew in blood cultures and the antibody titre against cytomegalovirus increased. The occurrence of septic diseases due to opportunistic microorganisms is a result of modern chemotherapy, advances in surgical instrumentation and the improvement of laboratory techniques for the detection of bacteria. These bacteremias often occur on the basis of side-effects of chemotherapy damaging cells with the development of pancytopenia. The host's predisposition is essentially rooted in malignant diseases, metabolic diseases and collagen diseases. A particularly serious threat are infections by multiple pathogens and endotoxic shock. Therapy can no longer be limited to antibiotics but includes, in toxic or pancytopenic (W.B.C. under 1,000) cases, the full utilization of all therapeutic possibilities of an intensive-care unit, and often isolation.

References

ALTEMEIER, W. A.: Gram-negative septicemia: a growing threat. Ann. Surg. **168**, 530—542 (1967).

BECK, E.: Proteus sepsis. Schweiz. med. Wschr. **92**, 1708—1711 (1962).

BLAIR, E., WISE, A., MACKAY, A. G.: Gram-negative bacteremic shock. J. Amer. med. Ass. **207**, 333—336 (1969).

BODEY, G. P., NIES, B. A., FREIREICH, E. J.: Multiple organism septicemia in acute leukemia. Arch. intern. Med. **116**, 266—272 (1965).

DANIELI, G., DALMONTE, P. R., MONTRONE, M.: Anwendung von Azathioprin bei chronischer Hepatitis. Münch. med. Wschr. **112**, 503—506 (1970).

DEICHER, H., FRICKE, R., KRULL, P.: Behandlung chronischer Bindegewebserkrankungen durch Cytostatika. Münch. med. Wschr. **112**, 506—514 (1970).

ENDERLIN, F., LEUTENEGGER, A., BURRI, C., GIGON, F. J.: Der Endotoxin-Schock in der Chirurgie. Ref. Kongreßdienst Laborat. Hausmann, St. Gallen, 1970, and Anaesthesiologie u. Wiederbelebung **50**, 60—73 (1970).

FINLAND, M., JONES, W. F., Jr., BARNES, M. W.: Occurrence of serious bacterial infections since introduction of antibacterial agents. J. Amer. med. Ass. **170**, 2188 (1959).

FREID, M. A., VOSTI, K. L.: The importance of underlying disease in patients with gram-negative bacteriemia. Arch. intern. Med. **121**, 418—423 (1968).

GARDNER, P., GRIFFIN, W. B., SHWARTZ, M. N., KUNZ, L. J.: Nonfermentative gram-negative bacilli of nosocomial interest. Amer. J. Med. **48**, 735—749 (1970).

GSELL, O.: Krankheiten durch Erreger der Mimea-Herellea-Gruppe. In: GSELL u. MOHR: Infektionskrankheiten, Bd. II, S. 676—681. Berlin-Heidelberg-New York: Springer 1968.

— Krankheiten durch Paracoli-Bazillen. In: GSELL u. MOHR: Infektionskrankheiten, Bd. II. Berlin-Heidelberg-New York: Springer 1968.

HERMANS, P. E., WASHINGTON, J. A.: Polymicrobial bacteremia. Ann. intern. Med. **73**, 387—392 (1970).

HOCHSTEIN, H. D., KIRKHAM, W. R., MAC YOUNG, V.: Recovery of more than 1 organism in septicemias. New Engl. J. Med. **273**, 468 (1965).

McCABE, W. R., JACKSON, G. G.: Gram-negative bacteriemia. Arch. intern. Med. **110**, 847—855, 856—864 (1962).

McHENRY, M. C., MARTIN, W. J., WELLMAN, W. E.: Bacteremia due to gram-negative bacilli. Ann. intern. Med. **56**, 207—219 (1962).

MEYER, W.: Klinik, Pathogenese und Therapie des Schockzustandes bei Sepsis durch gram-negative Erreger. Schweiz. med. Wschr. **96**, 137—143 (1966).

OECHSLIN, R., SCHEITLIN, W., FRICK, P.: Schockzustände bei Sepsis mit gramnegativen Erregern. Schweiz. med. Wschr. **92**, 1151—1155 (1962).

Prof. O. GSELL
CH-4000 Basel
Maiengasse 56

Discussion

SIEGENTHALER: I think Prof. GSELL generally agreed that in these conditions we can find septic complications. I would like to ask if you feel that today we have the obligation to start prophylactic chemotherapy when we use cytostatic therapy, or what would be the indication to start such treatment? This is a very difficult question and I should like to know if you can answer it?

GSELL: I would say that antibiotic prophylactic measures are not necessary in cancer chemotherapy as Prof. ERICSSON said because cytostatic therapy in cancer is an accepted treatment which you have to give today in nearly all cases. We must take into consideration that complications such as pancytopenia or bacteremia can develop. We must monitor the blood and when the WBC gets below 1000, specially the neutrophils; I believe that only then do we have to begin with antibiotic therapy. We must also control the bone marrow. By repeated blood cultures we determine the invasive strain and then start with intensive specific treatment. It is better not to begin with antibiotics early because you never know how long you have to continue and when you can finish because therapy with the cytostatics must be continued much longer than only a few days.

SIEGENTHALER: I feel the same as Prof. GSELL and Prof. ERICSSON but since newer investigations clearly show that prophylactic chemotherapy provides a better prognosis in these diseases, this question is not yet clearly answered.

GSELL: Another question is the prophylactic isolation of cancer patients with pancytopenic complications. In the United States, special isolation rooms are now being tested. It is difficult for us to arrange, for 1 or 2 such rare cases, strict isolation treatment, which is very expensive in personnel. There are always psychologic difficulties in such isolation. Also the results are problematic. Only if the WBC has dropped below 1,000 and you suspect a febrile bacteremia, does this seem to be the right moment to separate these patients and to institute isolation. The clinical conditions of the patient will determine what to do with regard to antibiotic therapy.

WILLIAMS: When the circulating white blood cells decrease, the bacteria from patient's own gut and skin invade. Experience suggests that isolation at the stage when the leucopenia develops is usually far too late to do any good in preventing the infective complications of immunosuppressive or cytotoxic therapy. In the patients whom we have seen with immunosuppression for renal transplantation, the infections developed have often been quite clearly shown to be with organisms that the patients were harbouring on or in their body in the week before the infection developed.

KASS: Along these same lines, we ought to try to define these conditions a little more precisely. First my own impression—and I wonder what Prof. GSELL thinks—is that the pancytopenia is not critical to the patient unless the count gets very low—that is—below a few hundred per cubic mm. Even patients with a thousand cells seem to do quite well clinically and certainly can mobilize an inflammatory leukocyte response locally. Second is this whole question of isolation. If the crucial feature is the gut bacteria then we certainly do not have a very convincing case. While I agree that many of our colleagues in the United States have published a great deal of information on this, I have yet to see useful information in terms of evaluating how really valuable this type of reverse precaution is in prolonging the life of a patient.

Gsell: I would like to ask Prof. Kass about corticosteroids; the question always raised in these cases: Shall we continue the corticosteroids? Their use stimulates the WBC and the thrombocytes, but favour also the appearance of bacteremia.

Kass: I think one has to say the answer is Yes. We must always consider whatever is being treated against the possible harm from corticosteroids, but in general they reduce resistance

Bayer-Symposium III, 157—163 (1971)
© by Springer-Verlag 1971

Influence of Antibiotic Treatment on the Bacterial Flora of Severe Burns

K. Wickman and H. Ericsson

With 6 Figures

For more than 15 years we have been interested in the infection of burns. We have studied the bacterial flora of burn wounds and of the hospital environment during the stay in hospital and during antibiotic treatment of severely burned

Table 1. *Staphylococcus aureus in the patients in relation to erythromycin-treatment*[a]

	Total number of patients	With resistant staphylococci[b]	With erythromycin-resistant staphylococci
Treated with erythromycin	2	2	2
Admitted before November 20, 1956	5	5	0
Admitted November 20, 1956, to January 30, 1957	6	5	5
Total	13	12	7

[a] Treatment period: November 20 to December 3, 1956.
[b] Resistant to one or more antibiotics other than erythromycin.

patients. This question becomes more and more pertinent as one has learned, to a great extent, how to bring these patients through the primary shock, but at a later stage the patients often succumb to secondary shock following generalized infections.

In 1957 in connection with erythromycin treatment of two patients with staphylococcal septicemia we found that erythromycin-resistant strains rapidly emerged and spread all over the ward. However, erythromycin-resistant staphylococci were not found in any of the patients already in the ward when the treatment started (Table 1). These patients were all heavily infected with other staphylococcal strains. All but one of the patients admitted within 10 weeks after the introduction of erythromycin were colonized by the resistant strains. It was thus found that the bacterial flora first established in the wounds could, to a certain extent, prevent colonization with the often more pathogenic and antibiotic-resistant bacteria present in the hospital environment.

                    K. WICKMAN and H. ERICSSON

These clinical observations could be documented by animal experiments (Fig. 1). Small third degree burns were produced in guinea pigs and inoculated with a strain of *Staphylococcus epidermidis* cultured from the animals' normal flora. These animals showed significantly less growth of *Staph. aureus* (sprayed upon the burns or spontaneously appearing) than control guinea pigs not inoculated with the interference strain.

The bacterial flora of 693 burned patients was studied during the two 5-year periods, 1954 to 1958 and 1962 to 1966. Some changes of treatment were made between the two periods, all of them probably affecting the more favourable

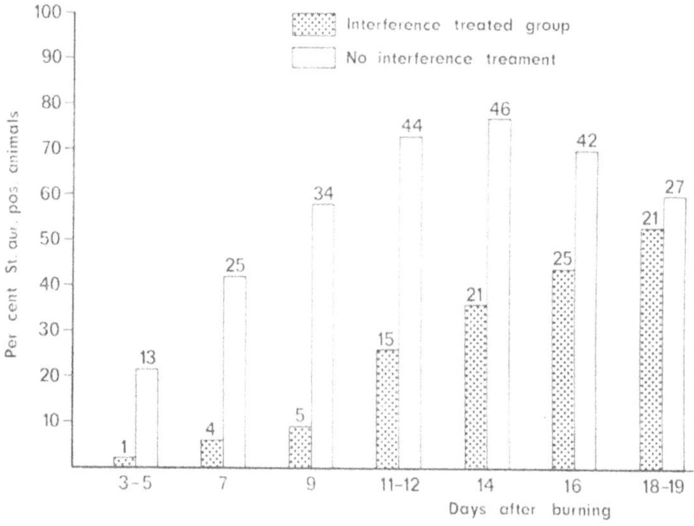

Fig. 1. Frequency of animals showing *Staph. aureus* in interference treated and non-treated groups at different times after burning. The figures above the columns denote number of positive animals

results in the later period, regarding mortality, hospitalization time and infection rate. Some of the observations made in these comparative studies could be interpreted in the light of the clinical and experimental observations of interference.

In the first 2 years of the earlier period, prophylaxis with penicillin or a combination of penicillin and streptomycin was given routinely to all burned patients. This prophylaxis was abandoned because it favoured the early colonization of the burns with resistant bacterial strains. Not even the incidence of beta-hemolytic streptococci was influenced because of the presence of penicillinase-producing staphylococci. The penicillinase-stable penicillins were not available at that time.

In the second period, prophylaxis was given only to patients with suspected or manifest pulmonary damage, or if hemolytic streptococci were present in the environment, including the patients own nose and throat (Table 2a). The prophylaxis in this period was given, in most cases, as a combination of benzyl-penicillin and a penicillinase-stable penicillin. Broad-spectrum antibiotics were given only in isolated cases. Unlike in the earlier period, there was no increase in the number of patients harbouring hemolytic streptococci in the wounds after prophylaxis. The incidence of *Staph. aureus* was not influenced, and the prophylaxis seemed rather to have a stimulating effect on Pseudomonas.

The effect on the flora of therapeutic use of antibiotics, usually after sensitivity testing on the bacteria found, was very good with the combined penicillin therapy

Table 2. *Influence of systemic treatment on the bacterial flora of the burn wounds, 1962 to 1966*

	No of patients	No of examined patients	β-hemolytic streptococci before after		*Staph. aureus* before after		Pseudomonas before after	
a) Prophylaxis								
Benzyl-penicillin	28 (25)	12	2	1	3	7	0	3
Penicillinase-stable penicillin	13 (11)	12	0	0	6	8	0	3
Benzyl-pc (or ampicillin) + penicillinase-stable penicillin	67 (62)	51	9	1	21	26	1	17
Other antibiotic alone	5 (4)	5	1	0	2	5	0	0
Penicillins + other antibiotic	1 (1)	1	0	0	1	1	0	0
Total	114 (103)	81	12	2	33	47	1	23
b) Therapy								
Benzyl-penicillin	25	20	12	6	16	13	0	3
Penicillinase-stable penicillin	16	15	4	0	12	5	1	8
Benzyl-pc (or ampicillin) + penicillinase-stable penicillin	57	51	27	0	43	18	4	13
Other antibiotic alone	37	24	3	0	14	19	9	9
Penicillins + other antibiotics	34	26	5	1	17	12	6	10
Total	169	136	51	7	102	67	20	43

Number in brackets indicate patients with extensive or medium-sized burns.

on hemolytic streptococci and rather good on *Staph. aureus* (Table 2b). The frequency of Pseudomonas was considerably higher after all kinds of therapy with penicillins as compared with the pretreatment flora and was not influenced by other antibiotics.

Comparing the changes of the bacterial flora between the two periods and in the individual patients during the course of the disease, gave the following results (Fig. 2): beta-hemolytic streptococci in the extensive burns showed a significant decrease during the latter period (1962 to 1966). There were few cross-infections that could be ascribed to these bacteria and systemic infections caused by

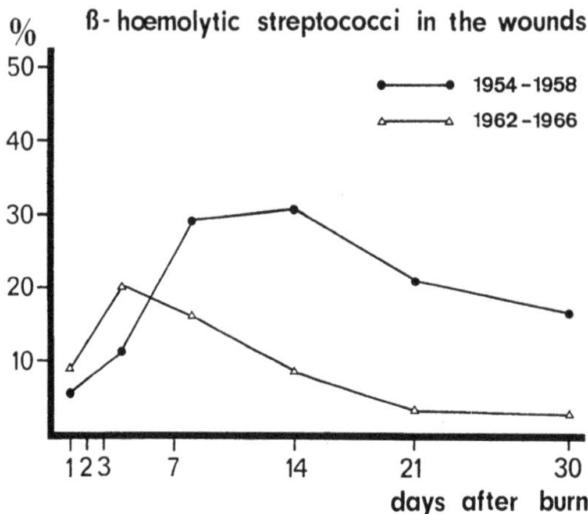

Fig. 2. Beta-hemolytic streptococci in the wounds

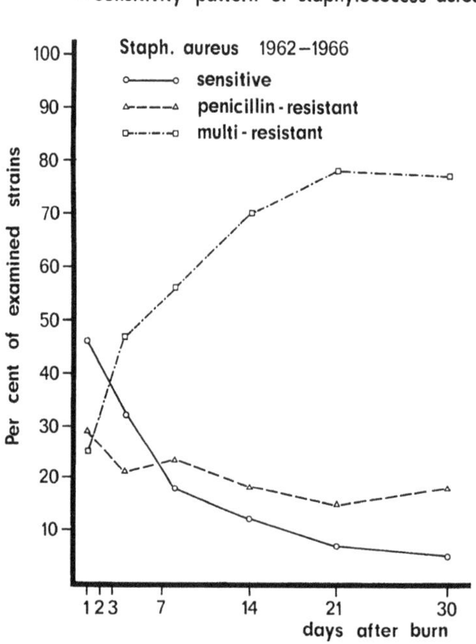

Fig. 3. Sensitivity pattern of *Staph. aureus* in the wounds (about 100 strains in each sampling)

streptococci were not seen. The combined penicillin-therapy probably played a part in this reduction.

The bacterial flora in the burns was dominated by *Staph. aureus* in both periods, but the number of severe systemic infections due to these bacteria decreased.

By studying the occurrence of *Staph. aureus* strains with different sensitivity patterns at different times after burning, it was found that totally sensitive strains dominated at the beginning, together with strains resistant only to benzylpeni-

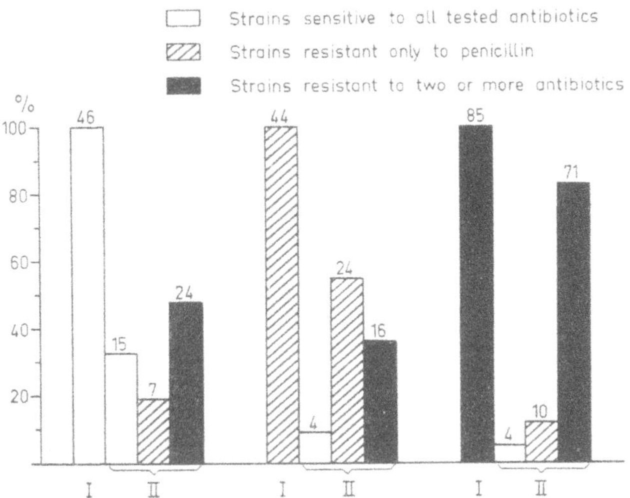

Fig. 4. Persistence of *Staph. aureus* with a given sensitivity pattern. The figures above the columns denote number of patients. I: First sampling. II. Later samplings

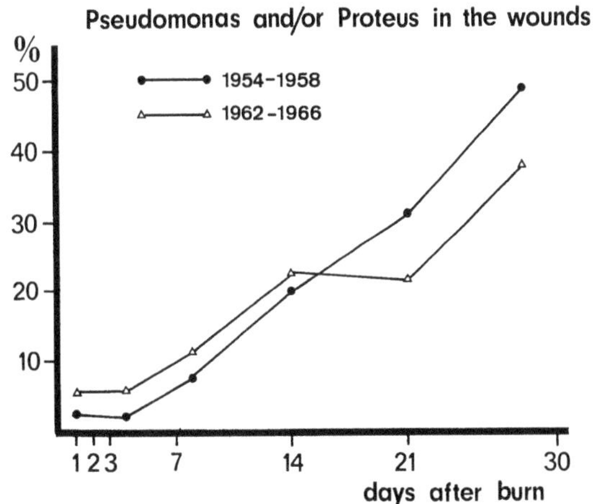

Fig. 5. Pseudomonas and Proteus in the wounds

cillin (Fig. 3). By the end of the first week, multi-resistant strains were already more common and after 3 weeks they reached a maximum of 78%.

In the patients with *Staph. aureus* in the wounds, it was found that the initial strains had a tendency to persist throughout the stay in hospital and, in particular, it was very rare that a resistant strain was replaced by one with greater sensitivity to antibiotics (Fig. 4).

Regarding the *gram-negative rods*, most reports from other countries tell about a considerable increase of gram-negative infections, especially with Pseudomonas (Fig. 5). We have not had the same experience in the Stockholm material and we believe that it is at least partially due to the restrictive use of chemo-prophylaxis, especially with broad-spectrum antibiotics. The only cases where gram-negative infections were more common during the later period were among the patients with bronchopneumonia. The patients with pulmonary burn injuries were almost the only ones who got antibiotic prophylaxis.

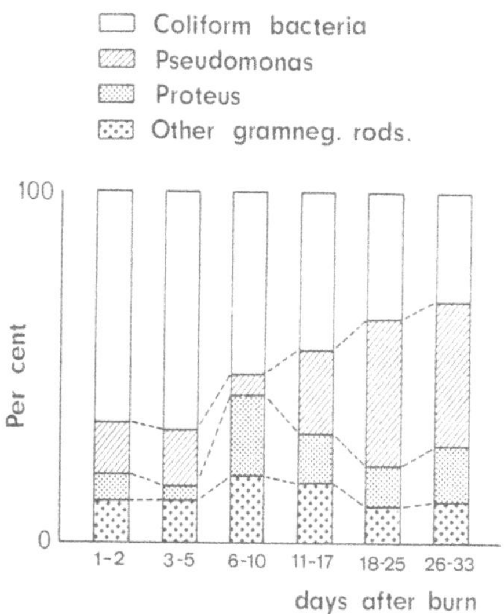

Fig. 6. Frequency of different types of gram-negative rods as a percentage of the total number of specimens with gram-negative rods at the given time after injury

The gram-negative rods are not very well suited for studying the change of sensitivity pattern, as they have often a naturally high resistance to several antibiotics. However, it was observed that the usually more sensitive coliform bacteria dominated during the first 10 days after injury, but from the end of the second week, Pseudomonas predominated (Fig. 6).

Some conclusions may be drawn from these observations. Careful and restrictive use of antibiotics under guidance of laboratory investigations is essential to:

obtain good therapeutic results in the individual patient;

avoid appearance and spread of resistant strains in hospitals;

preserve the efficacy and innocuousness of antibiotics.

These precautions are especially essential in the treatment of patients with severe burns, since inadequate antibiotic treatment could favour the invasion of the tissues by therapy-resistant bacteria at an early stage when the patient is extremely susceptible to infection because of the immuno-paralysis that constitutes a part of the primary shock syndrome.

Prof. Dr. H. Ericsson
Bacteriological Department
Karolinska sjukhuset
S-104 01 Stockholm 60

Discussion

Finland: Do you use the terms "multiple resistant" and "methicillin-resistant" synonymously ?

With respect to your inverted umbrella that becomes a funnel, I recall in the early days—I think a surgeon in Britain named Chalmers, talked about "operatting ander an umbrella of antibiotics". At that time I used the term "seive" instead of umbrella. With the increase in the number of antibiotics one uses, one just increases the size of the holes on the mesh of the seive, the size of the mesh being proportional to the resistance to the strains that come through.

Ericsson: May I answer your first question. By multiple resistance we mean resistant to more than penicillin and we do not mean methicillin-resistant strains, because we have not observed any. As to the question about the appeerence of pseudomonas infections after treatment with stable penicillins, my opinion is that this is an effect of the general rule of etiological effects. There are some strains of Pseudomonas around in any hospital, and probably in any large unit. It is only if they are given the favourable situation that their competitors —other bacteria—are eliminated that they are then able to establish themselves as infecting agents. That is why we take the attitude that you should not be changing all bacteria around the hospital. In the patient there are some bacteria in bones. We believe that Staphylococcus is a good example where the patient gets along rather well and it does not matter so much if he has them. What you do with antibiotics, in my opinion, is that you cannot eliminate the infections, you can only change the etiology. Therefore, my presentation here is, to some extent, an answer to the question which is the main subject of this whole meeting. Much of the change in etiology in the individual case and, in the long run, in the hospital is caused by antibiotics and can be avoided by not using antibiotics.

As to the special question of staphylococci, I would like to mention two observations which seem to some extent contradictory. One is that patients harbouring staphylococci in their wounds, in which clinician regards the infection as not important at all, because he has, for instance, been able to get his skin grafts to grow well. Meanwhile the patient himself has been fighting these bacteria —if you allow the expression—because he has been producing antistaphylolysin, I am not of the opinion that the mere appearance;—colonisation and some pus.

and so on, in the bones is of importance in the infection. I much prefer the gram-positive to the gram-negative infection and think we can avoid the gram-negatives by just leaving the gram-positives alone.

CHABBERT: I should like to ask a question of Prof. ERICSSON. If we determine the MIC of a Pseudomonas to carbenicillin, generally Pseudomonas appears sensitive to carbenicillin, except maybe in a very low percentage of strains harbouring R factors—harbouring (A) characters (penicillinase production), in my own experience such types represent only 1% or 2% of the strains. Such strains are resistant to 10,000 µg of carbenicillin per ml. It might be interesting to know if in patients with burns, such kinds of high resistance of Pseudomonas with R factors might be found?

GSELL: From your picture with the umbrella, is it not best to change this umbrella? That is to say, use a limited, interrupted therapy, then wait for a time. Do you know when these activities are changed and when to use another? That is my question.

ERICSSON: May I first answer the question of Prof. GSELL. We have not tried this but I know that this system was used, for instance, by the late Mary Barber at the Hammersmith Hospital and with some success. We have not found it necessary to try it because we are rather satisfied with our results. As to Dr. CHABBERT's question, I would emphasize that the material dates from two periods, 1954 to 1958 and from 1962 to 1966; carbenicillin and the information which you give me now, were not available at that time so they have not been studied.

DASCHNER: Prof. ERICSSON, do you have figures comparing the outcome in patients receiving prophylactic treatment and in those receiving no antibiotic treatment?

ERICSSON: These are the two periods which have been described in detail here in the booklet which I shall be happy to send you. There has been a decrease of mortality. To what extent this can be ascribed to the lack of, or to the omission of antibiotic therapy and to what extent it can be ascribed to non-specific treatment, which consists mainly of administration of blood, albumin and gamma globulin, and which has been exchanged for what previously was routine, I cannot say. I would also add that the latest new method that has been introduced in the burns unit is that relating to the observations that such patients have a very high basal metabolism—they lose very much heat through their burn wounds. Now, all extensive burns are put under a fan blowing hot air so that they do not lose the heat but they, of course, lose a lot of fluids, and this has to be replaced. This has had a very favourable effect on the treatment, as I have mentioned in my introduction. These were just examples of a new type of treatment and are not included in this material at all.

Bayer-Symposium III, 165—171 (1971)
© by Springer-Verlag 1971

An Antibody Response in Pyelonephritis after Change in Causative Organisms

W. MARGET

With 4 Figures

The question of antibody response (ABR) in repeated infections with different microorganisms is one of interaction between bacteria, that is, the antigenic changes within a single species or the interplay of the antigenic composition of multiple species. These conditions can be observed in chronic pyelonephritis of children. In this model we are presented with an opportunity for specific bacterial diagnosis, analysis, good antibody response and, moreover, a group in which relapse after treatment or superinfection is a common occurrence.

We recently reported that the leucocyturia is without relevance in relation to the antibody response (MANTEL et al.).

The following questions seem important to us in the antibody response:

1. Does a decrease or an increase of the antibody titer occur after a long period of disease ?

2. Do different groups produce different antibody levels with and without obstructive urinary tract infection (UTI) ?

3. Is the antibody titer modified in a double infection and, if so, in which respect ?

4. Are the number of changes of causative organisms related to different antibody levels ?

Materials and Methods

Patients. The following report is based on 25 cases of chronic pyelonephritis in children. The study lasted over a period of about 3 years. Ten children suffered from an obstructive form of pyelonephritis, the remaining 15 were without primary abnormalities of the urinary tract. The first ten patients were children with uropathy associated with obstruction or a neurogenic bladder. The persisting bacteriuria may have two causes: the first one is an increasing bacterial growth in bladders with insufficient function, as shown with Fairley's method of "washout", as a proximally located obstruction, and the second is probably a lack of tissue function of the mucous membrane or parenchyma of the urinary system.

The symptoms of disease in the patients are characterized by the disappearance of the tested and treated organisms, with a relapse of significant bacteriuria with one or two other organisms after a few days. Sometimes the etiology of the relapse is clear when it can later be demonstrated that the different strain of bacteria was present before therapy.

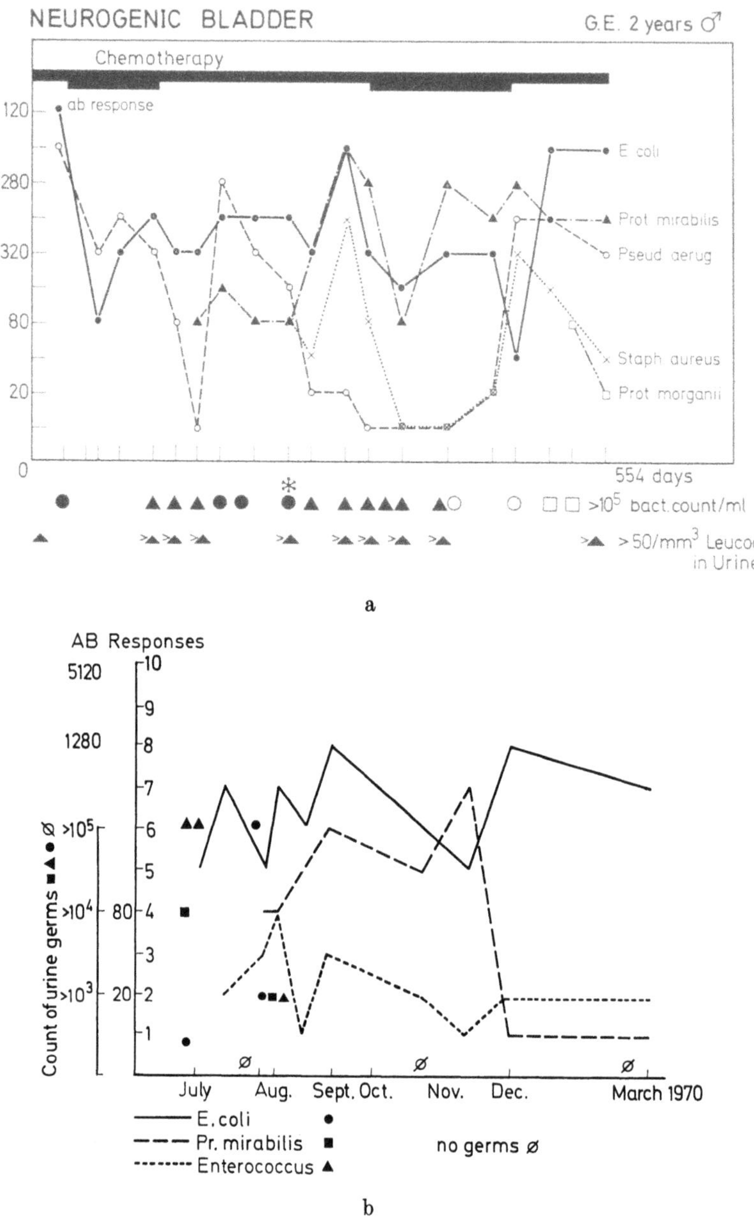

Fig. 1a and b. ABR in changing infections in chronic pyelonephritis

In other cases the occurrence of a new strain after therapy cannot be explained, but sometimes after a second change of treatment, the first causative organism reappears, therefore, it was still present but not isolated.

Antibody Determination. First we have to mention one defect in our investigation, but this is not a serious one. We made no serologic identification of isolated strains of *E. coli*. It seemed unnecessary because we use the homologous *E. coli* in every test. Since in this species there is a broad cross antigenicity, we cannot demonstrate changes from one strain of *E. coli* to another. A modification of the method of BADER, described by NETER, was used for hemagglutination titrations. The range of normal titers was obtained with a pooled antigen (ANDERSON), which indicates the highest possible ABR against types of the *E. coli* group in about 95% (FLAMM et al.).

A titer increase after a change in the bacteria was considered significant under the following conditions:There must be an increase of at least two or more steps of titer. If there are two enterobacteriaceae with a probable common antigen, for example, *E. coli*, Klebsiella, Proteus, we accepted only an increasing titer, if the

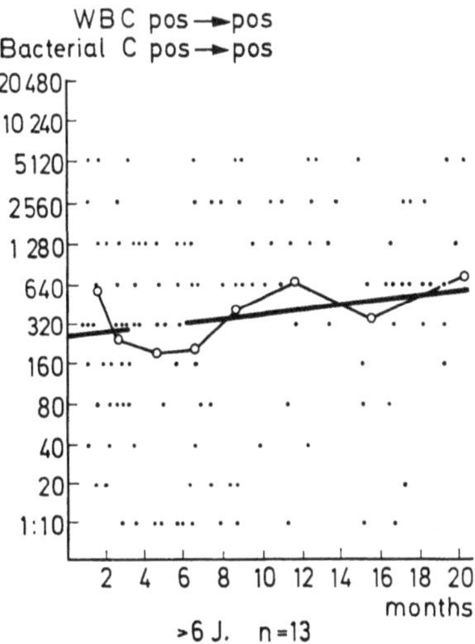

Fig. 2. ABR in chronic pyelonephritis under constant conditions (pathologic WBC and changing significant bacteriuria)

strain yielding the increased titer should cross react with the other similar-reacting strain and only when the titer obtained with the earlier strain either decreased or remained stationary (Figs. 1 a and b).

The first question about the behaviour of the ABT is answered by Fig. 2, which contains some cases in which significant bacteriuria persisted. These titers together show a slight increase in the regression line. This observation demonstrates that there is no decrease in the humoral antibody response, but also no extremely marked reaction, in spite of the continuous stimulation by the antigens. Fig. 3 shows the regression line *E. coli* titers decreasing while those of the titers of other bacteria rises. On the other hand, there is no failure of antigen build-up nor exhaustion by these humoral antigens.

As previously noted, we separated our patients into two groups, the first included children with findings after obstruction, either with or without prior operation, and the other group with no abnormalities. This differentiation was made because it was felt that there may be a different immunologic behaviour in the two groups which probably affects the change in the causative organisms and in the ABR.

Both groups were observed over an average of about 2 years (Table 1). Only significant bacteriuria or a positive culture after suprapubic bladder punction was considered. Two children, one in each group, had significant bacteriuria continuously with no clear relations between ABR and urinary tract infection.

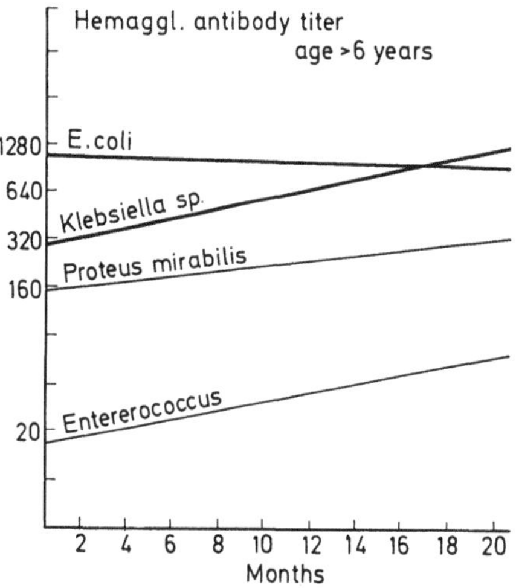

Fig. 3. Regression lines of different bacteria in pyelonephritis

Table 1. *Changes of causative organisms in pyelonephritis (PN)*

Number of	Obstructive PN	Not obstructive PN
Cases	10	13
Controls (investigation)	195	267
Months	251	281
Changes	31	55

The periods of observation were nearly the same in both groups, nevertheless, we found under the same therapeutic conditions, a different number of changes in the isolates (Table 2).

The ABR after a change in the infection seems to show another difference. In the non-obstructive group the AB titers rose in nearly three quarters of the cases, whereas in the other group there were fewer rises (Table 3).

Our results show that a double infection is certainly possible. But we observed that this was not the rule and that other possibilities were more often seen. There

Table 2. *The frequence of isolation of changed bacteria in pyelonephritis (PN)*

	Obstructive PN	Nonobstructive PN
1. Controls per month	0.8	1
2. Controls per change	6	5.2
3. Months per change	8	5

Table 3. *Change of causative organism and AB response (ABR) in pyelonephritis (PN)*

	Obstructive PN	Nonobstructive PN
With ABR	11	22
Without ABR	6	8
	17	30
ABR without changes of bacteriuria	18	16

Table 4. *Double infection and AB response in pyelonephritis (PN)*

	Increase of AB titer	
	Obstructive PN	Nonobstructive PN
None	0	4
One	2	5
Both	0	2
	2	7

were many cases where there was significant bacteriuria with single organism without a rise of antibody titer; there were other cases where there was an increasing antibody titer and the corresponding or another strain with a similar antigenicity was not isolated, and finally there was a "real" double infection without antibody reaction to either of the infecting strains. In particular, ABR in children with obstructive disease was seldom observed (Table 4).

Conclusions

A relation of the titer to the frequency of change in the causative organisms in urinary tract infections (significant bacteriuria) was not detected. It seems to depend on the alternating of therapy with the frequency of regular observations in the patients. However, in our opinion, it depends mainly on the kind of abnormalities in the urinary tract and on a damage in parenchyma of the kidney and mucous membrane or parenchymal tissue.

One point of view not previously noted seems remarkable to us: The titer of antibody to *E. coli* always shows a smaller tendency to decrease after elimination of the *E. coli*. That might be an important difference (Fig. 1a and b). The children

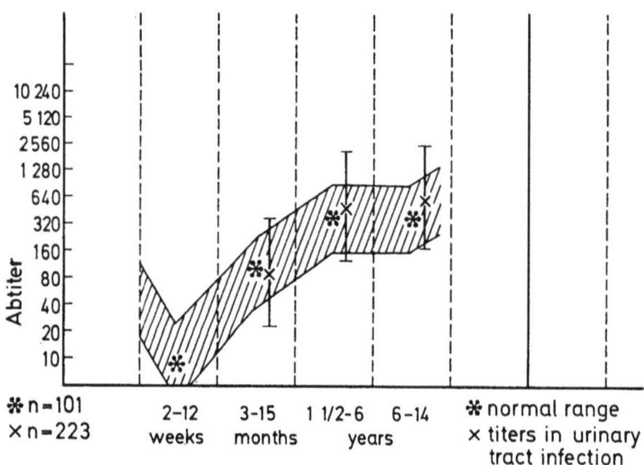

Fig. 4. ABR of *E. coli* in chronic pyelonephritis compared with the range of normal titers of a pooled antigen in different age groups

with chronic pyelonephritis showed no increase or decrease at all in the range of titers of *E. coli* (Fig. 4).

We confirmed the observation that there is no detectable interference between different infecting strains, probably even in a triple infection. The response of stimulating humoral antibodies in this severe chronic disease seems to be normal or, under specified conditions, impossible to establish.

A good antibody response is of no importance for the prognosis of chronic pyelonephritis, but we can not be quite sure of this since we had our patients under regular antibiotic control. From our investigations, based on the criteria of high antibody titers, we believe that urinary tract infections in children without obstructive abnormalities involved the kidney more often than in infected obstructive uropathies.

References

ANDERSEN, H. J.: Studies of urinary tract infections in infancy and childhood. J. Pediat. **68**, 542 (1966).
BADER, R.-E.: (Pers. communication, 1970).

FLAMM, U., MARGET, W.: Beeinflußt die Aristol ochiasäure-Behandlung den Antikörpertiteranstieg bei chronischer Pyelonephritis? In: LOSSE, H., KIENITZ, M.: Die Pyelonephritis. Stuttgart: Thieme (im Druck).

MANTEL, K., MARGET, W., DASCHNER, F.: Harnweginfektionen ohne Harnbefunde. Mschr. Kinderheilk. 118, 324 (1970).

NETER, E.: Bacterial hemagglutination and hemolysis. Bact. Rev. 20, 166 (1956).

Prof. Dr. W. MARGET
Abt. für antimikrob. Therapie
Univ.-Kinderklinik München
D-8000 München
Lindwurmstraße 4

Discussion

KASS: I am delighted that Prof. MARGET and his associates are looking into this important problem and am pleased to hear emphasised what the field has not always learned, namely, the overwhelming importance of non-obstructive disease. The excessive emphasis on the problem of obstruction has kept us from understanding chronic pyelonephritis and the present data have supported the growing indication that obstruction is only a small part of the problem, and it is this type of study that is needed.

One other factor that is important is the use of the homologous strain for the antibody determinations. Dr. ELDER and I have published comparative studies in which large numbers of patients were following with a battery of the most commonly occurring E. coli serotypes, comparing the titres obtained with these strains with titres to homologous strains. Always the patient's infecting strain gave higher antibody titres than did the common serotypes.

The haemagglutinin reaction is excessively dependent on IgM. We know that IgM is more likely to produce haemagglutination by a factor of 50 to 100, as compared with IgG. As the ratio of IgM/IgG changes there may be an apparent decrease in titre when the total amount of antibody has, in fact, risen. Dr. ZINNER and I are looking at this problem using indirect fluorescence. As one might anticipate, there are many patients, particularly the more chronic ones, who get surprisingly high IgG titres and the IgM titres do not reflect this. For example, patients with chronic urinary infection and hypertension seem to have IgG titres that are exceedingly high and there is no reflection of this in the haemagglutinin titres. One additional small point is not clear from the data, and that is the matter of "significant bacteriuria" in children. We have great difficulty in establishing bacteriuria in children because the rates of contamination are so high, and we are unhappy about trusting any simple culture, no matter how high the count. We prefer two or three consecutive cultures to show the same organism before we are ready to accept high counts as meaningful.

MARGET: Thank you very much. I agree with you completely. We repeated our investigations too. If we are not sure that there is significant bacteriuria in any case, we do a suprapubic bladder puncture. That is the only way to clear it up and we try to get out what is necessary as to what the IgA titre means in this connexion.

FINLAND: Any other questions for discussion—is anyone interested in the urine, Dr. KASS.

KASS: There are a few patients with IgA and IgG in the urine. At the moment no pattern has emerged which allows us to put special significance to these findings.

Bayer-Symposium III, 173—188 (1971)

L-Forms: Problems and Outlook

F. D. Daschner, V. Jouja and B. M. Kagan

With 11 Figures

The problems with L-forms began when Klieneberger in 1935 isolated a strange organism from a culture of *Streptobacillus moniliformis*. She designated it as L1 and considered it to be a symbiotic mycoplasma strain. For many years the bacterial forms of the streptobacilli obscured the true identity of their accompanying L-forms until Dienes in 1938 uncovered the secret and showed that these pleomorphic forms were not mycoplasmas but were derived from the bacterium itself.

At present we have a vast amount of theoretical knowledge and information which can be found in several excellent reviews and books (Crawford et al., 1966; Guze, 1968; Hayflick, 1969; Feingold, 1969). Many investigators, however, accompanied their new contribution with a new name, so that today we read about L-forms, L-phase bacteria, bacterial variants, cell wall defective bacteria, protoplasts and spheroplasts (referring to the same or different things). For this presentation we shall use the following definitions: "L-forms" are bacteria without a rigid cell wall, their morphology, mode of reproduction and structure of colonies are altered and are similar to those of pleuropneumonia-like organisms (PPLO). The absence of that part of the cell wall that gives rigidity to the bacterium explains most of the properties of L-forms, such as pleomorphism, colonial morphology, filterability, mechanical and osmotic fragility. "Protoplasts" are bacteria without any cell wall whatsoever. "Spheroplasts", on the other hand, are osmotically fragile bacteria, which retain parts of the cell wall structure.

Protoplasts and spheroplasts may assume the colonial morphology of L-form colonies when grown on L-form media. The amount and the production of cell wall material in L-forms and spheroplasts varies considerably (Kandler et al., 1958, Hofschneider et al., 1968).

Stable L-forms grow in the absence of an inducing agent and do not revert, whereas unstable L-forms revert to the bacterial form when the inducing agents such as a penicillin, cephalosporin, glycine or lysozyme are removed from the medium. The inducing agents have in common the property of either preventing the formation of the murein sacculus of the bacterium or dissolving already existing murein. The transition of a bacterium into the L-form is accompanied by marked changes in the requirements for cultivation. These requirements are serum, low concentrations of agar and a high content of sucrose or salt or some other substance to provide the so-called "osmotic stabilization" of the culture medium.

On an osmotically stabilized medium, L-forms grow as a small round colony with a dark center. This is due to the penetration in the center of densely packed granules of varying size into the agar, surrounded by a clear flat zone consisting of large round bodies of varying size on the surface of the agar, often referred to as the typical "fried egg" appearance of L-form colonies (Fig. 1).

Because of the ability of L-forms, induced by antibiotics, to revert to the bacterial form after removal of the inducer, clinically oriented investigators became aware of the possible importance of L-forms as a factor in chronic or relapsing infections, after Dienes and Smith (1944) first reported on the isolation

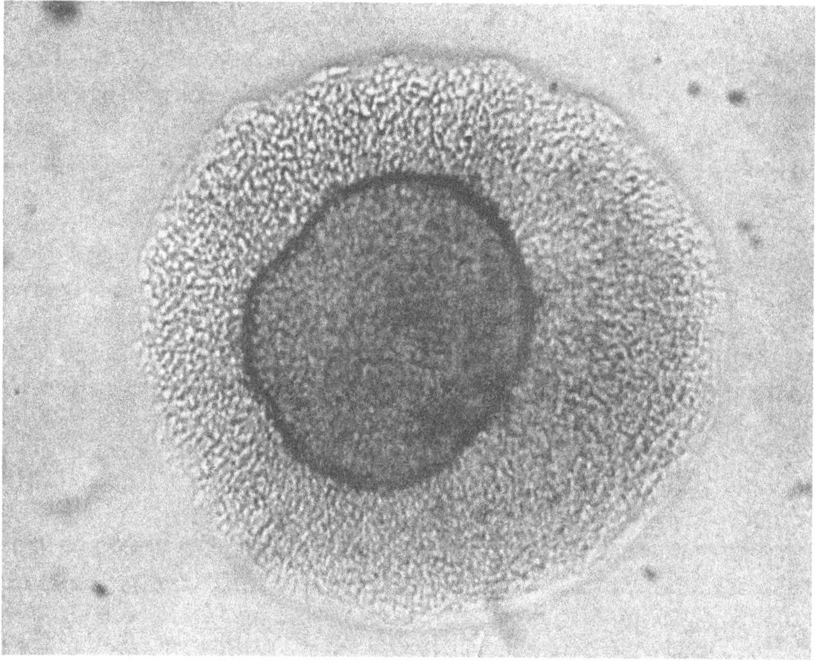

Fig. 1. L-form colony of *Proteus mirabilis* on salt-serum-agar after 3 days of incubation. The so-called "fried-egg" appearance is due to growth into the agar (dark central area). Unstained wet agar preparation, light micrograph (× 120 magnifiaction)

of an L-form from a patient. Today many *in vitro* and *in vivo* studies support the following hypothesis (Fig. 2):

(1) Many bacteria can be induced *in vivo* and *in vitro* to L-forms (spheroplasts or protoplasts) by various antibiotics (penicillin, cephalosporin, D-cycloserine, bacitracin, vancomycin, ristocetin), lysozyme, certain aminoacids (glycine), antiserum and complement, with or without the action of lysozyme (Lederberg, 1956; Weibull, 1953; Repaske, 1956; Godzeski et al., 1965; Mortimer, 1965; Kagan et al., 1962; Muschel, 1968; Wittler, 1952; Landman et al., 1958; Hayflick, 1969).

(2) Bacteria as L-forms (spheroplasts or protoplasts) change their structure, antigenicity(?), pathogenicity, biochemical properties and sensitivity to anti-

microbial agents. They survive *in vivo* and *in vitro* and can be isolated from animal and human sources.

The L-form per se is generally not pathogenic even when it derives from a pathogenic bacterium. KLIENEBERGER (1938) noted that "mice could not be infected by the L-forms of *Streptobacillus moniliformis* which itself was pathogenic". KLIENEBERGER (1938), DIENES (1951) and later several other investigators (WITTLER, 1952; FREUNDT, 1956) noted, however, that when unstable

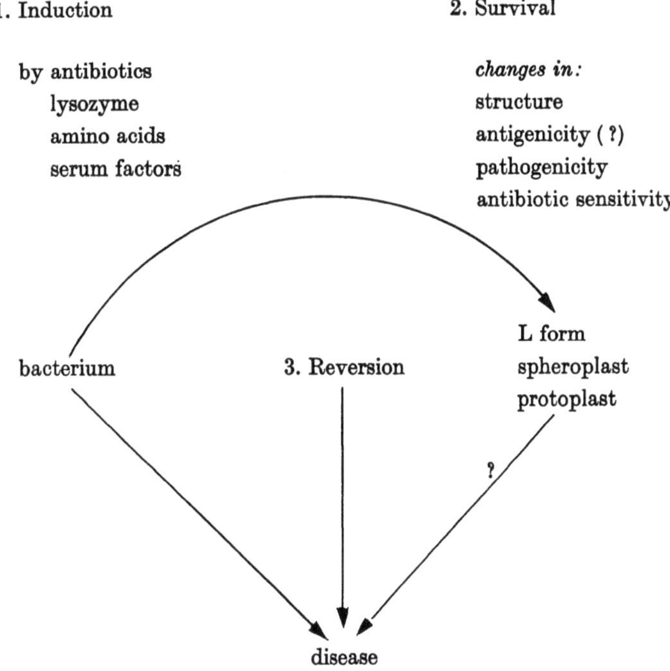

Fig. 2. Possible role of L-forms in recurrent infections

L-forms reverted in the experimental animal to bacterial forms the bacteria were again pathogenic. However, it is not yet possible to state definitely that pathogenic L-forms do not exist (KAGAN, G. Y., 1968). Recently McKAY et al. (1966) reported that intratracheal instillation of a stable "protoplast" form of *Haemophilus parainfluenzae* in pigs resulted in pneumonia in all cases. "Protoplasts" were seen and isolated from the pulmonary lesions. The ability of L-forms to revert *in vivo* to pathogenic bacteria and the fact that some L-forms produce endotoxin (KALMANSON et al., 1968) and exotoxins (SCHEIBEL et al., 1959; MADOFF et al., 1961) in amounts approximately equal to that produced by the bacterial forms, suggest that L-forms have at least disease-producing potential.

Immunologic studies in experimental animals revealed antigenic differences of streptococcal L-forms as compared to the bacterial forms (LYNN et al., 1968).

Whether or not L-forms can initiate pathologic lesions in man, based on immunologic mechanisms needs investigations.

Of clinical importance are the differences in the antibiotic sensitivity patterns
of L-forms from those of their "parent" bacteria (Kagan et al., 1964; Teuber,
1969). L-forms are resistant to the penicillins and cephalosporins; staphylococcal
L-forms are more sensitive to polymyxin B, aminoglycoside antibiotics and
erythromycin, oleandomycin, lincomycin and tetracycline.

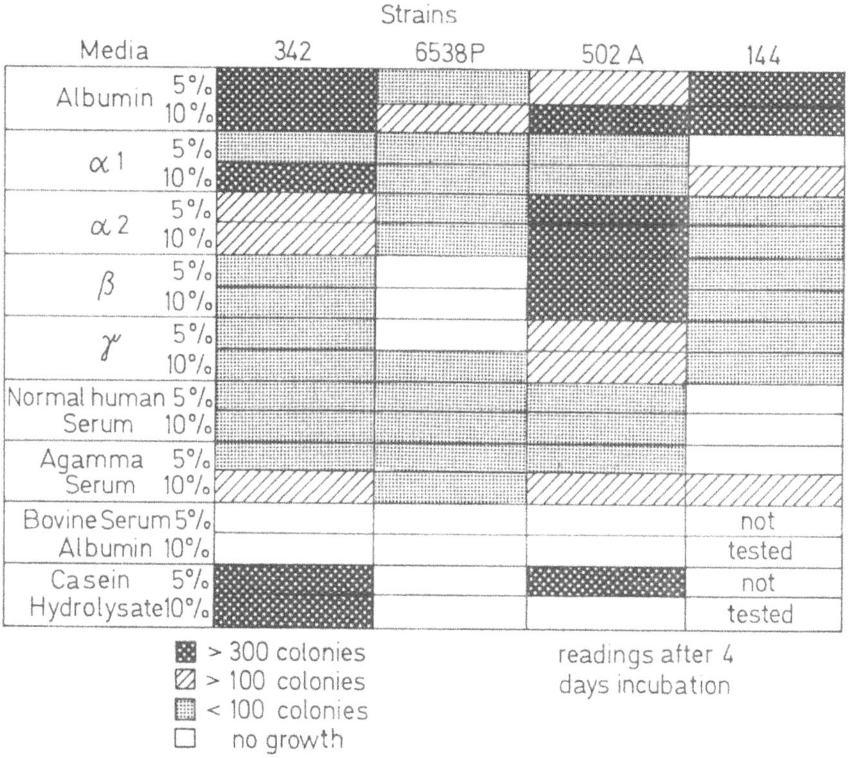

Fig. 3. Comparison of growth of L-forms from four different staphylococcal strains after
4 days of incubation on salt-serum-agar containing 5 or 10 % of various sera, proteins or serum
protein fractions

(3) Under special circumstances, such as omission of the inducing agent,
L-forms and spheroplasts revert in vivo and in vitro to the bacterial form (Taubeneck et al., 1955; Freundt, 1956; Winterbauer et al., 1967).

It is beyond the scope of this presentation to discuss in detail the studies on
clinical isolation of L-forms which are reviewed in several recent articles (Hayflick, 1969; Feingold, 1969). Two methods are generally employed to isolate
L-forms and to separate the L-form from the bacterial form. Specimens are
cultured in control medium and in osmotically stabilized medium or filtered

through a filter that retains the bacterial phase. If classical bacteria grow only on the hypertonic medium inoculated with the specimen itself or the filtrate of the specimen, one may be dealing with reverted L-forms or spheroplasts; if the organisms grow as typical L-form colonies, the isolation of L-forms is on a firm basis. The isolation procedure, however, is complicated by several factors: passage of L-forms through filters results in considerable loss of viable elements (VAN BOVEN et al., 1968): the growth of staphylococcal L-forms is inhibited by the corresponding

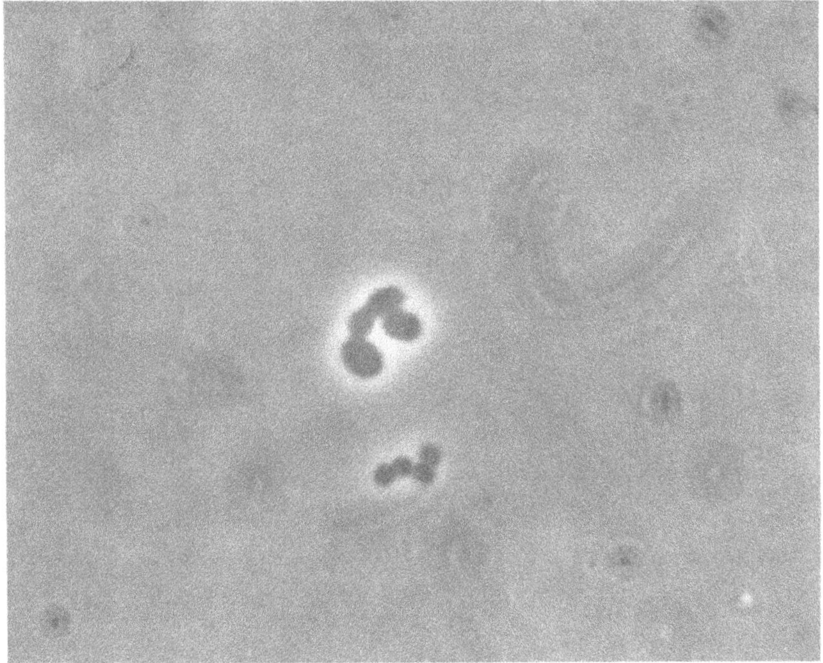

Fig. 4. Staphylococcal spheroplasts in various stages of development (above) and normal staphylococci (below), in salt-serum-broth after 1 day of incubation. The strain was isolated from a patient with chronic osteomyelitis (case No. 3 in Table 1). The spheroplasts were filtrable through a 0.45 µ Millipore filter and reverted to staphylococci within 24 h on osmotically stabilized salt-serum-agar, but not on brain heart infusion agar

coccal form (KAGAN, CHR. et al., 1969), and L-forms of different organisms grow best on different media (LANDMAN et al., 1958). We even found considerable differences in the growth of four strains of stable staphylococcal L-forms on media containing various proteins and serum protein fractions (Fig. 3) (JOUJA et al., unpublished data). Four strains of staphylococcal L-forms were inoculated on salt-serum-agar containing 5 or 10% of nine different proteins or serum protein fractions. The growth was determined by the number of colonies after 4 days of incubation at 37 °C. The inconsistent results, even among strains of one bacterial species, demonstrates the peculiar growth and protein requirements of L-forms. In general, however, higher concentrations of albumin, α_1- or α_2-globulin, and agamma serum enhance the growth better than normal human serum.

One of the principle interests of our laboratory, as far as clinical isolations are concerned, was the isolation of staphylococcal L-forms from sputum of patients with cystic fibrosis (KAGAN, 1968); 33 of 116 cultures revealed L-forms of staphylococci. In addition to these findings we isolated L-forms (unpublished data), identified morphologically by the Dienes' technique (MADOFF et al., 1967), or

Table 1. *Isolation of L-forms and osmotically fragile bacteria from clinical material. Summary of cases*

Case	Patient, age, diagnosis	Isolation of L-form	Osm. fragile bacteria	Normal bacteria	Material	Antibiotic therapy 2 months prior or during the L-form isolation
1	M. P., $1^1/_2$ months, myelomonocytic leukemia		Staphylococcus	Staphylococcus	Thymus	no
2	L. O., 14 years, brain abscess		Staphylococcus	no	Pus	yes
3	M. B., 10 years, chronic osteomyelitis		Staphylococcus	Staphylococcus	Pus	no
4	L. G., 4 years, chronic urinary tract infection	*Ps. aeruginosa*		*Ps.aeruginosa*	Urine	yes
5	R. D., 40 years, chronic osteomyelitis	*Proteus mirabilis*		*Proteus mirabilis*	Pus	no
6	P. T., 4 years, chronic urinary tract infection	*E. coli*		*E. coli*	Urine	yes

osmotically fragile bacteria which grew only on osmotically stabilized media, but not on routine control media from thymus, in 1 case of congenital leukemia, from urine in 2 cases of relapsing urinary tract infections, from pus in one brain abscess and in 2 cases of osteomyelitis (Table 1). In 5 of 6 cases, the bacterial forms were also found; 5 of 6 L-forms were isolated from pus or urine, both providing osmotic protection to osmotically fragile bacteria or L-forms.

Antibiotic therapy (even therapy with an antibiotic which acts on the cell wall) seems not to be necessary for the induction or survival of L-forms *in vivo*. In three of the 6 cases no antibiotic treatment had been given for at least 2 months prior to isolation of the L-form.

In case No. 3, staphylococcal spheroplasts in various stages of development could be demonstrated in salt-serum-broth by phase contrast microscopy (Fig. 4). These spheroplasts were filtrable and reverted to staphylococci on salt-serum agar but not on brain heart infusion agar. In case No. 5 spheroplasts from *Proteus mirabilis* could be induced in salt-serum-broth by 1 IU penicillin G/ml. These were morphologically indistinguishable from the clinically isolated spheroplasts. Fig. 5 shows that penicillin G-induced spheroplasts of *Proteus mirabilis* are highly susceptible to concentrations of polymyxin B sulfate (100 µg/ml) to which the rod form was resistant.

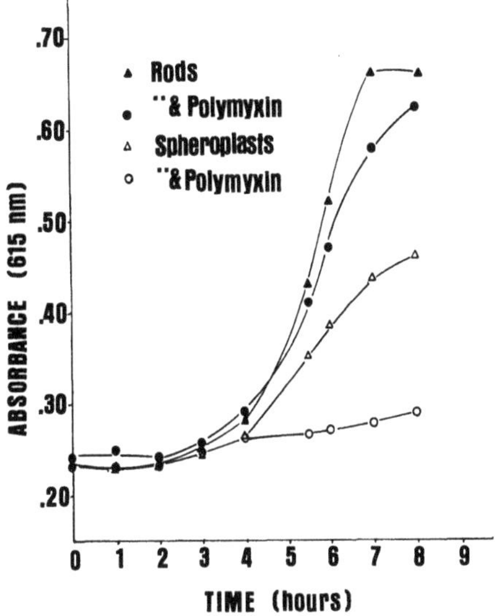

Fig. 5. Susceptibility to polymyxin B sulfate (100 µg/ml) of rods and penicillin G- induced spheroplasts (1 IU/ml) of *Proteus mirabilis,* isolated from a patient with chronic osteomyelitis (case No. 5 in Table 1). Growth curves were obtained by hourly measurements of the optical density with a Coleman Jr. Spectrophotometer

Pyelonephritis is the disease in which the theoretical basis for the survival of L-forms or spheroplasts and their possible role as persisters has been most extensively studied (BRAUDE et al., 1962, 1968; ALDERMAN et al., 1963; GUTMAN et al., 1965, 1968; GNARPE, 1970 (1); GNARPE et al., 1970 (2); KALMANSON et al., 1968), because the hypertonic renal medulla and urine are a protective environment for these osmotically fragile bacteria. We investigated the morphologic changes in a strain of *Proteus mirabilis,* isolated as an unstable L-form and normal rod from a patient with chronic osteomyelitis, under the influence of penicillin in normal human urine (DASCHNER et al., unpublished data).

Bacteria from an overnight culture of *Proteus mirabilis* in trypticase soy broth (BBL) were inoculated into sterile fresh urine with different osmolalities and penicillin concentrations (buffered potassium penicillin G) to a final concentration of 10^{8-9}/ml and incubated at 37 °C. Fig. 6a—h shows the transformation of rods

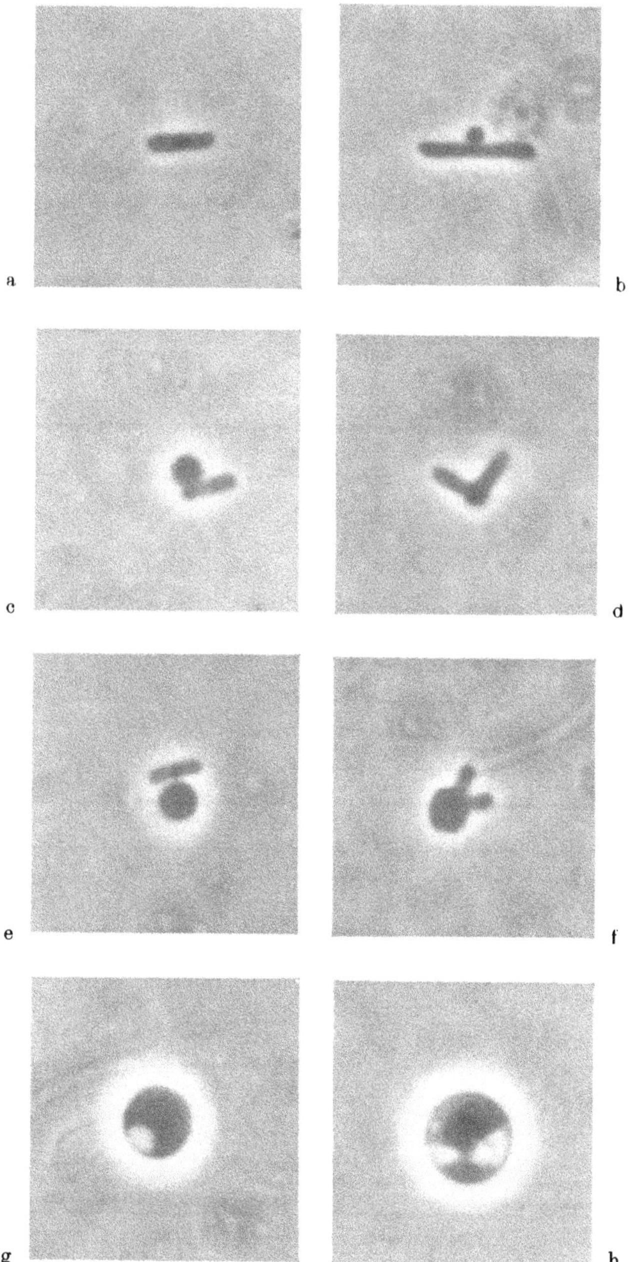

Fig. 6. Morphologic changes in a rod of *Proteus mirabilis* during induction to transitional forms (b—f), small (g), and large (h) spheroplasts in hypertonic human urine by 100 IU penicillin G/ml (× 1,840 magnification, phase contrast microscopy)

into spheroplasts. This induction process takes about 1 to 2 h. A swelling originates at the end or the center of the bacterium which gradually increases in size, "absorbs" the remainder of the rod (Fig. 6f) and finally becomes an absolutely round, small spheroplast (Fig. 6g). Since penicillin inhibits the crosslinking of mucopeptide chains and mucopeptide is the only cell wall component taking part in the initial

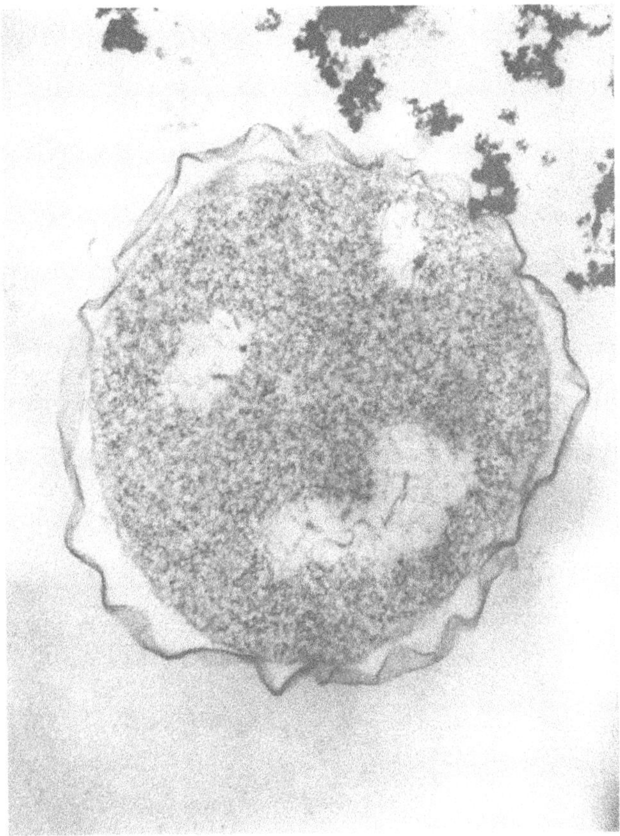

Fig. 7. Electron micrograph of a sectioned spheroplast induced in *Proteus mirabilis* by peni-cillin G in urine. Section shows finely granular protoplasm surrounded by well defined cyto-plasmic membrane and highly folded, nonrigid cell wall. Densities in upper left of micrograph represent urinary salt crystals (× 35,000 magnification)

stages of septum formation and cell division, the weakening of the cell wall struc-ture shows first in polar or central areas of the bacterium (MURRAY, 1968).

Electron microscopic studies have shown that the spheroplasts which were induced in urine are still surrounded by a non-rigid cell wall resembling the "unstable spheroplast L-form" of *Proteus mirabilis* described by HOFSCHNEIDER et al. (1968) (Fig. 7). Most small spheroplasts develop to large spheroplasts by

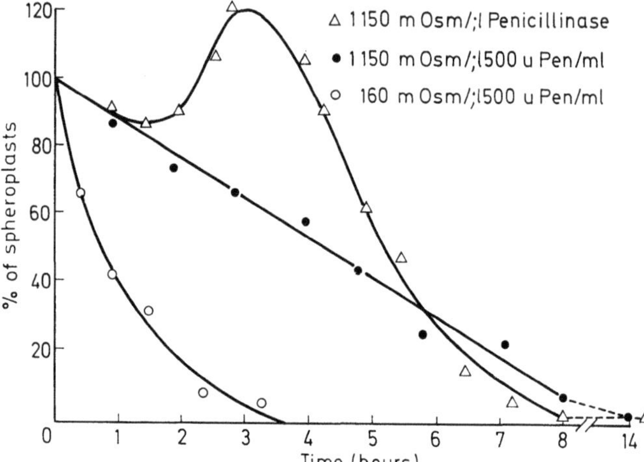

Fig. 8. Survival of spheroplasts in hypertonic (1,150 milliosmal/l) and hypotonic (160 milli-osmol/l) urine. Spheroplasts lyse in hypotonic urine more rapidly than in hypertonic urine containing 500 IU penicillin G/ml. Inhibition of penicillin by penicillinase increases the number of spheroplasts by division for about 2 h in hypertonic urine. Penicillinase was added at the beginning of the experiment. Spheroplasts were counted in a bright light hemocytometer, the number of surviving spheroplasts was recorded as percent of the number present at time "0". Since Ca and Mg ions are necessary for stabilization of spheroplasts, the precipitation of urinary salts was prevented by adjusting the pH of the urine between 5.5 and 6.5 with 0.1 N HCL

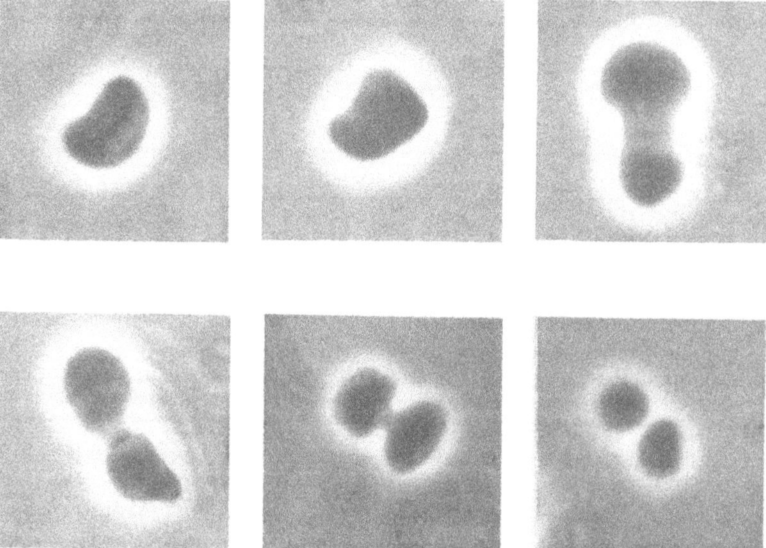

Fig. 9. Division of penicillin G-induced spheroplasts in urine by constriction and binary fission after addition of penicillinase. Due to loss of a rigid cell wall, spheroplasts change their shape during the division process which takes 50 to 60 min (× 1,840 magnification, phase contrast microscopy)

increasing the diameter up to 80% (Fig. 6h). If 0.1 ml of the spheroplast culture
was inoculated in salt-serum-agar pour plates, numerous ordinary colonies of
Proteus mirabilis grew after 12 to 24 h incubation; after 48 to 72 h several typical

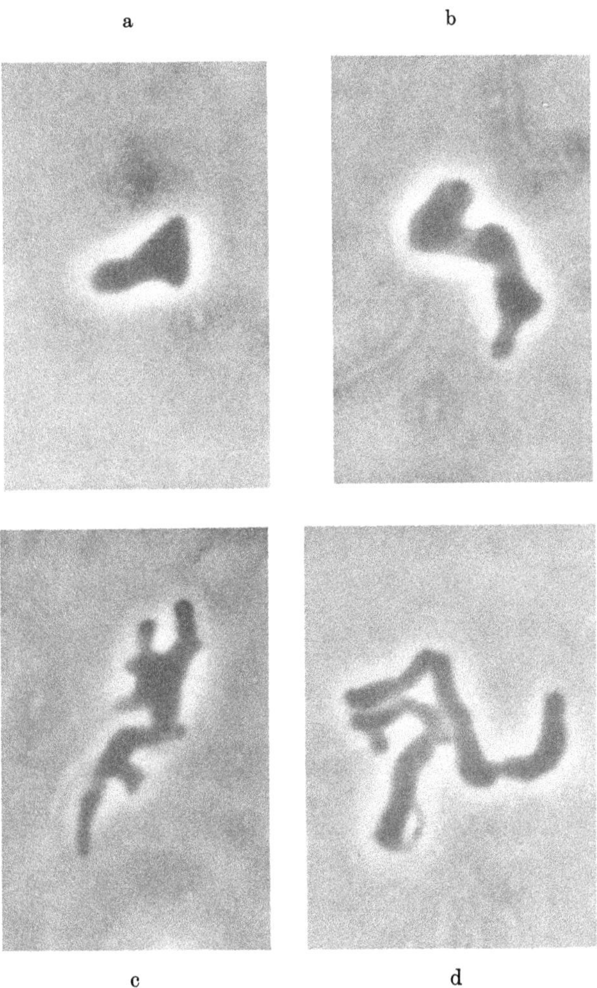

Fig. 10. Reversion of spheroplasts of *Proteus mirabilis* in urine to normal rods by elongation
(a), branching (b, c) and segmentation (d, e). One spheroplast sometimes generates up to
20 rods (f, g). Reversion starts 30 to 60 min after addition of penicillinase and takes 3 to 4 h
(×1,840 magnification, phase contrast microscopy)

L-form colonies appeared, which subsequently reverted completely over a period
of 1 to 2 days. Spheroplasts inoculated in hypo-or hypertonic urine containing
either penicillinase or 500 IU penicillin G/ml lysed within 3 to 4 h in hypotonic
urine, but were preserved much longer in hypertonic urine (Fig. 8). Up to 8%
were still present after 8 h incubation; after 14 h all spheroplasts were either lysed

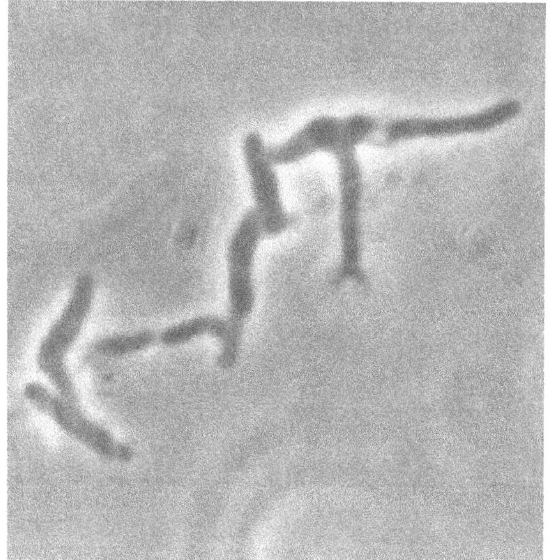

e

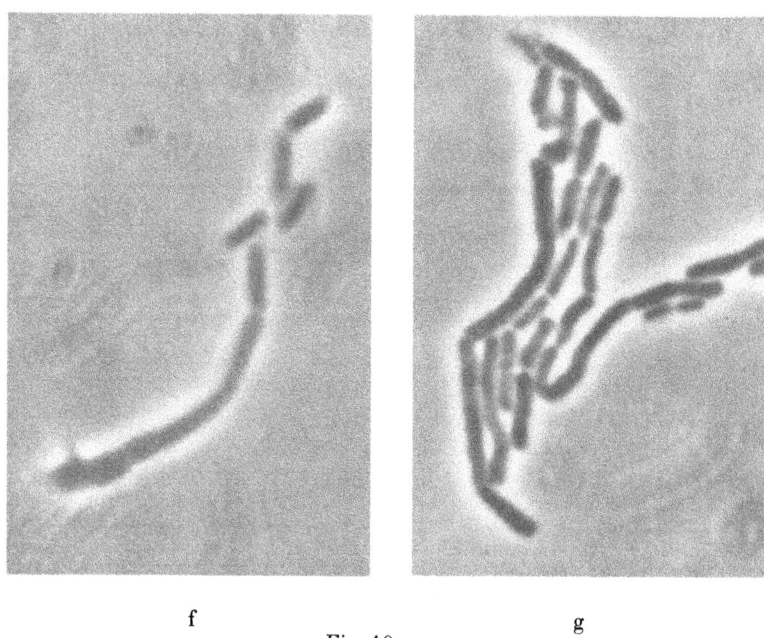

f   g

Fig. 10 e—g

or in the process of lysis in urine containing penicillinase; 0.5% were surviving in urine with penicillin. If the action of penicillin was inhibited by penicillinase, most spheroplasts started to revert or to divide at this high osmolality, causing a remarkable increase in their number after 1 to 2 h, which exceeded the number originally present. The rapid fall of the survival curve after 3 to 4 h is partly caused by lysis, but to a greater part by reversion.

Division of spheroplasts in urine starts 30 to 60 min after addition of penicillinase and takes 50 to 60 min. Each spheroplast gives rise to two equally sized round or ellipsoid spheroplasts formed by constriction and binary fission (Fig. 9). Fig. 10a—g illustrates several consecutive steps of the reversion process which almost invariably starts from large spheroplasts after addition of penicillinase. This process involves three mechanisms-elongation, branching and segmentation The spheroplast first elongates (Fig. 10a) then develops amoeboid filamentous

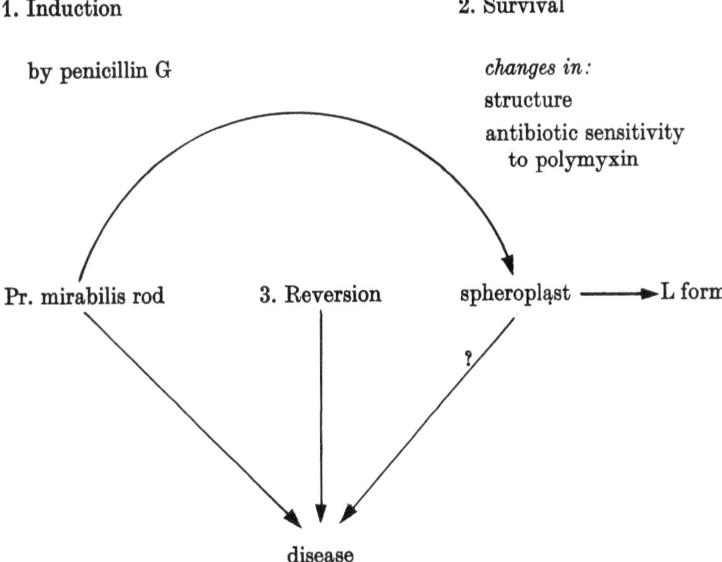

Fig. 11. Possible role of *Proteus mirabilis* spheroplasts as persisters in recurrent urinary tract infections

projections (Fig. 10b), which appear at several places around the periphery at the same time (Fig. 10c); the branches elongate further, and finally segment to large rod like forms (Fig. 10d, e). Several divisions break the rod-like forms into typical motile rods (Fig. 10f), so that one spheroplast sometimes generates up to 20 rods (Fig. 10g). The whole step takes 3 to 4 h. The number of dividing and reverting spheroplasts seems to depend mostly upon the osmolality of the urine. Up to 80% started to revert at 1,200 milliosmol/l (10 to 20% completed the reversion process); only 5 to 10% started to revert at 450 milliosmol/l; no reversion occurred at 160 milliosmol/l.

Similar morphologic changes of bacteria under the influence of penicillin *in vitro* have been described before (DIENES, 1949; TAUBENECK et al., 1955; LIEBERMEISTER et al., 1956; STEMPEN et al., 1951; MEDILL et al., 1954). To our knowledge ours is the first study which provides morphologic evidence that penicillin G-induced spheroplasts of *Proteus mirabilis* are able to grow, divide and survive in hypertonic urine over a considerable period of time. In rat kidney, L-forms and protoplasts have been shown to survive much longer (Braude et al., 1968; Kalmanson et al., 1964). The ability of spheroplasts to revert to normal bacterial form after removal of the antibiotic inducer may play a role in recurrence or persistence of chronic bacterial urinary tract infections (Fig. 11).

The outlook for L-form research is still not clear. Thirty-five years of intensive work in this field have not answered to one most vital question which clinicians continue to ask: „What is the biological and clinical significance of L-forms of bacteria ?". By inprovements in our definitions, isolation techniques, media and interpretation of results we may be able to convince bacteriologists and clinicians, that bacteria are at least as smart in surviving hostile conditions as we are to produce them.

References

Alderman, M. H., Freedman, L. R.: Experimental pyelonephritis. X. The direct injection of Escherichia coli protoplasts into the medulla of the rabbit kidney. Yale J. Biol. Med. 36, 157—164 (1963).

van Boven, C. P. A., Ensering, H. L., Hijmans, W.: Size determination by the filtration method of the reproductive elements of group A streptococcal L-forms. J. gen. Microbiol. 52, 403—412 (1968).

Braude, A. J., Siemienski, J.: Production of bladder stones by L-forms. Trans. Ass. Amer. Phycns 81, 323—333 (1968).

— — Jacobs, J.: Protoplast formation in human urine. Trans. Ass. Amer. Phycns 74, 234 to 245 (1962).

Crawford, Y. E., Smith, P. F., Panos, Ch., Lynn, R. J.: A microbial enigma. Myoplasma and bacterial L-forms, 1st. ed. Cleveland and New York: The World Publishing Co. 1966.

Dienes, L.: Further observations on the L organism of Klieneberger. Proc. Soc. exp. Biol. (N.Y.) 39, 365—367 (1938).

— The development of Proteus cultures in the presence of penicillin. J. Bact. 57, 529—546 (1949).

— Smith, W. E.: The significance of pleomorphism in bacterioides strains. J. Bact. 48, 125 to 153 (1944).

— Weinberger, H. J.: The L-forms of bacteria. Bact. Rev. 15, 245—288 (1951).

Feingold, D. S.: Biology and pathogenicity of microbial spheroplasts and L-forms. New Engl. J. Med. 281, 1159—1170 (1969).

Freundt, E. A.: Experimental investigations into the pathogenicity of the L-phase variant of Streptobacillus moniformis. Acta path. microbiol. scand. 38, 246—258 (1956).

Gnarpe, H.: Spheroplast infections of the urinary tract. Scand. J. infect. Dis. 2, 59—64 (1970).

— Edebo, L.: Conditions affecting the viability of spheroplasts in urine. Infect. Immun. 1, 300—304 (1970).

Godzeski, C. W., Brier, G., Griffith, R. S., Black, H. R.: Association of bacterial L-phase organisms in chronic infections. Nature (Lond.) 205, 1340 (1965).

Gutman, L. T., Turck, M., Petersdorf, R. G., Wedgwood, R. J.: Significance of bacterial variants in urine of patients with chronic bacteriuria. J. clin. Invest. 44, 1945—1952 (1965).

— Winterbauer, R. H., Turck, M., Wedgwood, R. J., Petersdorf, R. G.: The role of bacterial variants in experimental pyelonephritis. In: Guze, L. B.: Microbial protoplasts, spheroplasts and L-forms, 1st ed., pp. 391—395. Baltimore: The Williams and Wilkins Co. 1968.

Guze, L. B.: Microbial protoplasts, spheroplasts and L-forms, 1st ed. Baltimore: The Williams and Wilkins Co. 1968.

Hayflick, L.: The Mycoplasmatales and the L-phase of bacteria, 1st. ed. New York: Appleton-Century Crofts 1969.

Hofschneider, P. H., Martin, H. H.: Diversity of surface layers in L-forms of Proteus mirabilis. J. gen. Microbiol. 51, 23—32 (1968).

KAGAN, B. M.: Role of L-forms in staphylococcal infection. In: GUZE, L. B.: Microbial protoplasts, spheroplasts and L-forms, 1st ed., pp. 372—378. Baltimore: The Williams and Wilkins Co. 1968.
— MOLANDER, C. W., WEINBERGER, H. J.: Induction and cultivation of staphylococcal L-forms in the presence of methicillin. J. Bact. 83, 1162—1163 (1962).
— ZOLLA, S., BUSSER, R., LIEPNIEKS, S.: Sensitivity of coccal and L-forms of *Staphylococcus aureus* to five antibiotics. J. Bact. 88, 630—632 (1964).
KAGAN, CHR., JANEFF, J., KAGAN, B. M.: Inhibition of L-forms of staphylococci by coccal forms of staphylococci. Proc. Soc. exp. Biol. (N.Y.) 132, 807—808 (1969).
KAGAN, G. Y.: Some aspects of investigations of pathogenic potentialities of L-forms of bacteria. In: GUZE, L. B.: Microbial protoplasts, spheroplasts and L-forms, 1st ed., pp. 422—443. Baltimore: The Williams and Wilkins Co. 1968.
KALMANSON, G. M., GUZE, L. B.: Role of protoplasts in pathogenesis of pyelonephritis. J. Amer. med. Ass. 190, 1107—1109 (1964).
— KUBOTA, M., GUZE, L. B.: Production of the Shwartzman reaction with microbial L-forms. J. Bact. 96, 646—651 (1968).
KANDLER, O., HUND, A., ZEHENDER, C.: Cell wall composition in bacterial and L-forms of *Proteus vulgaris*. Nature (Lond.) 181, 572—573 (1958).
KLIENEBERGER, E.: The natural occurrence of pleuropneumonia-like organisms in apparent symbiosis with *Streptobacillus moniliformis* and other bacteria. J. Path. Bact. 40, 93—105 (1935).
— Pleuropneumonia-like organisms of diverse provenance: Some results of an inquire into methods of differentiation. J. Hyg. (Camb.) 38, 458—476 (1938).
LANDMAN, O. E., ALTENBERG, R. A., GINOZA, H. S.: Quantitative conversion of cells and protoplasts of *Proteus mirabilis* and *Escherichia coli* to the L-form. J. Bact. 75, 567—576 (1958).
LEDERBERG, J.: Bacterial protoplasts induced by penicillin. Proc. nat. Acad. Sci. (Wash.) 42, 574—577 (1956).
LIEBERMEISTER, K., KELLENBERGER, E.: Studien zur L-Form der Bakterien. I. Die Umwandlung der bazillären in die globuläre Zellform bei Proteus unter Einfluß von Penicillin. Naturforsch. 11 b, 200—206 (1956).
LYNN, R. J., HALLER, G. J.: Bacterial L-forms as immunogenic agents. In: GUZE, L. B.: Microbial protoplasts, spheroplasts and L-forms, 1st ed., pp. 270—278. Baltimore: The Williams and Wilkins Co. 1968.
MADOFF, M. A., MADOFF-ANNENBERG, S., WEINSTEIN, L.: Production of neuraminidase by L-forms of *Vibrio cholerae*. Proc. Soc. exp. Biol. (N.Y.) 107, 776—777 (1961).
MADOFF, S., BURKE, M. E., DIENES, L.: Induction and identification of L-forms of bacteria. Ann. N.Y. Acad. Sci. 143, 755—759 (1967).
McKAY, K. A., ABELSETH, H. K., VANDREUMEL, A. A.: Production of an enzootic-like pneumonia in pigs with "protoplasts" of *Haemophilus parainfluencae*. Nature (Lond.) 212, 359—360 (1966).
MEDILL, M. A., HUTCHINSON, W. G.: The reversion of the L-form of *Proteus mirabilis* into the rod form. J. Bact. 68, 89—92 (1954).
MORTIMER, E. A.: Production of L-forms of group A streptococci in mice. Proc. Soc. exp. Biol. (N. Y.) 119, 159—163 (1965).
MURRAY, R. G. E.: Bacterial cell wall anatomy in relation to the formation of spheroplasts and protoplasts. In: GUZE, L. B.: Microbial protoplasts, spheroplast and L-forms, 1st ed., pp. 1—18. Baltimore: The Williams and Wilkins Co. 1968.
MUSCHEL, L. H.: The formation of spheroplasts by immune substances and the reactivity of immune substances against diverse rounded forms. In: GUZE, L. B.: Microbial protoplasts, spheroplasts and L-forms, 1st ed., pp. 19—29. Baltimore: The Williams and Wilkins Co. 1968.
REPASKE, R.: Lysis of gram-negative bacteria by lysozyme. Biochim. biophys. Acta (Amst.) 22, 189—191 (1956).
SCHEIBEL, J., ASSANDRI, J.: Isolation of toxigenic L-phase variants from *Clostridium tetani*. Acta path. microbiol. scand. 46, 333—338 (1959).

Stempen, H., Hutchinson, W. G.: The formation and development of large bodies in *Proteus vulgaris* OX-19. J. Bact. **61**, 321—335 (1951).

Taubeneck, U., Mueller, M. R.: Über kontinuierliche Beobachtung des Formwandels von *Proteus vulgaris* unter Penicillineinfluß. Zbl. Bakt., I. Abt., Orig. **163**, 309—312 (1955).

Teuber, M.: Susceptibility to polymyxin B of penicillin G-induced *Proteus mirabilis* L-forms and spheroplasts. J. Bact. **98**, 347—350 (1969).

Weibull, C.: The isolation of protoplasts from *Bacillus megaterium* by controlled treatment with lysozyme. J. Bact. **66**, 688—702 (1953).

Winterbauer, R. H., Gutman, L. T., Turck, M., Wedgwood, R. J., Petersdorf, R. G.: The role of penicillin-induced bacterial variants in experimental pyelonephritis. J. exp. Med. **125**, 607—618 (1967).

Wittler, R. G.: The L-form of *Haemophilus pertussis* in the mouse. J. gen. Microbiol. **6**, 311—317 (1952).

Dr. F. Daschner
Cedars-Sinai Medical Center
Dept. Pediatrics, University of California.
Los Angeles (Director: B. M. Kagan)
4833 Fountain Avenue
Los Angeles, Cal 90029 (U.S.A.)

Bayer-Symposium III, 189—196 (1971)
© by Springer-Verlag 1971

Role of Deficient Mutants in Microbial Persistence

Y. A. Chabbert, Ph. Cayeux, and J. F. Acar

With 3 Figures

Microbial persistence, as defined by Walsh McDermott, is the capacity of a drug susceptible organism to survive drug attack when subsisting in an animal body. Microbial persistence takes place during treatment but it may be stable after treatment for a variable period of time: days, months or sometimes years. This persistent state is demonstrated by relapses due to a bacterium which has the same characteristics as the one causing the previous infection, with essentially the same so-called drug sensitivity. Persistence may also be discovered by isolating bacteria from the site of infection, for example, during surgery of a focus. Open cardiac surgery for replacing aortic valves in patients after apparent cure of streptococcal endocarditis is a good example of our present ability to check the eradication of Streptococcus, or conversely, to isolate persisting bacteria.

Pathogenic bacteria able to persist in the site of infection after the "curative" effect of chemotherapeutic agents might be considered to behave as organisms of low pathogenicity or as non-pathogenic for the patient during the persistent state.

Microbial persistence may consequently be considered as belonging to the wide range of conditions related to the low pathogenicity of bacteria. Drug sensitive bacteria persisting in the focus of infection during or after treatment no longer grow at the exponential growth rate. To be "drug indifferent" or to be able to "play dead" as McDermott termed it, bacteria have to modify their behaviour under the pressure of the drug and/or the environment in the host. In a general way the persistent state may be considered to be the result of a bacterial variation. Two types of bacterial variation have been defined: the phenotypic and genotypic; one or both may be observed in bacterial persistence.

A phenotypic variation is a non-hereditary change due to the environment in the host, the capacity of a bacterial cell to divide depending on the medium. In any medium the bacterial population reaches a maximum and division stops. *In vivo*, many factors limit the growth: physical conditions, metabolites, specific or non specific immunity. Bacteriological examinations of pathological products show that the number of bacteria or groups of bacteria, or bacterial microcolonies are not really increasing during the disease. Such limitations of growth directly influence the effect of antibiotics.

Antibiotics act poorly on slowly growing bacteria and on resting cells with low metabolic activity. Phenotypic change may lead to an anatomic defect, as in the case of unstable L-forms. These points are well known and have been extensively described. When the bacterial variation involved is phenotypic, a change in the environment conditions, such as the isolation from a pathological product in laboratory media, restores the full characteristics of the strain which was invading at the beginning of the infection.

However, this phenotypic variation is not the only one to be observed in bacterial persistence, genotypic variations may occur. Among the numerous mutants occurring spontaneously in a large bacterial population, the environment at the site of infection of treated patients may select two types of mutants. The first one—drug resistant mutants, are easily recognised *in vitro* by a stable significant increase in the minimum inhibitory concentration (MIC) of the selecting drug. These biochemical mechanisms of the various types of resistance are not all exactly defined but it is generally assumed that they are related to the primary site of action of the antibiotic, to permeability or to destroying enzymes.

The second is a large group of mutants which are still "sensitive" to the drug *in vitro* but able to survive *in vivo* under hostile conditions, including drugs. Such mutants are deficient in some process causing them to behave as "drug indifferent". Cell wall deficient variants (stable L-forms, type A), studied for many years (Guze) and responsible for bacterial persistence in clinical cases (Louria et al.) might be considered as an example of such deficiency. But it is not the only type of deficient bacteria able to persist *in vivo;* other stable variants exist which are not cell wall-deficient, as are the stable L-forms.

A very interesting category is represented by variants deficient in some metabolic pathway. Such variants also called *auxotrophic mutants*, have been extensively studied in genetics and in molecular biology. It is likely that environ mental conditions occurring *in vivo* in treated or non-treated patients are able to select many of them. A good example was recently reported by Cayeux et al. as thiol-requiring mutants of Streptococcus. One of their strains was isolated in the following conditions:

From a patient with bacterial endocarditis, a *Streptococcus lactis* group N (strain GAN) was first isolated; this group represent only 0.1% of strains studied in the laboratory (Wahl and Cayeux). The patient had been treated with penicillin G (50 mU/day) intravenously and streptomycin (1 g/day) i.m. for 20 days. Because of increasing cardiac failure, an aortic valve replacement was performed 2 weeks after stopping treatment. A Streptococcus (strain GAD) was isolated from the ground-up aortic valve. This Streptococcus was able to grow only as numerous small satellite colonies around a few colonies of the original strain (GAN); it could not grow on brain-heart-infusion (BHI) agar supplemented by serum or sucrose (20%) under aerobic or anaerobic conditions but was able to grow in BHI supplemented by thioglycollic acid and l-cysteine or glutathione. Only reducing agents containing the thiol group were able to promote the growth of this organisms to the same extent as the original strain of Streptococcus. In addition, by using penicillin for the selection of auxotrophic mutant, it has been possible to select, in two steps, a mutant with the same thiol requirements. For these reasons the strain of Streptococcus (GAD), isolated from the valve was considered to be a mutant of the *Streptococcus lactis*, group N (GAN) that initially infected the patient.

The purpose of our experiment was to compare, in an experimental model *in vivo*, the effect of antibiotics on streptococci belonging to groups D and N with thiol-requiring streptococcus, isolated by Cayeux et al.

Material and Methods

a) Strains

Streptococcus group D strain AL. CLA 0501; Streptococcus group N strain GAN N 51; Streptococcus group N thiol requiring GAD N 52.

b) Minimum Inhibitory Concentration in vitro

Agar dilution method—using Steers-like replicator. Inoculum: 10^4 to 10^5 bacteria per spot.

c) Experimental Model

Principle: As in bacterial endocarditis, bacteria are represented by microcolonies located in a fibrin clot. We tried to reproduce this situation by an agar disc containing growing colonies of *Streptococcus* inserted in the peritoneal cavity of mice. This method, derived from WERNER et al. was previously described by CHABBERT et al.

Inoculum: 0.1 ml of 10^{-3} dilution of 24 h broth culture containing 10^7 bacterial per ml is inoculated into 25 ml fresh rabbit blood, BHI agar (Difco) and poured in a Petri dish (9 cm). After solidification, a cylinder of agar (6 mm diameter and 4 mm high) is cut out with a cork borer. Each agar cylinder contained approximately 5 colony-forming units (CFU).

Insertion in peritoneal cavity of mice: Swiss mice (20 g) are laparotomized under ether anesthesia and two discs are inserted, one in each side of the peritoneal cavity; 20 mice are used per treatment.

Counting bacteria: At 2 day intervals, or at various other intervals, four agar discs are removed from two mice, ground in BHI broth and colony forming units counted by the dilution method on BHI agar supplemented by fresh rabbit blood. The number of CFU (bacteria) per disc are recorded.

Treatment

Dosage: Benzathine penicillin G (Specia-Paris) 10,000 U streptomycin (Specia-Paris) 5 mg, subcutaneously, twice a day for 15 or 20 days.

Onset of treatment: In studies on bacterial persistence, preliminary experiments showed that persistence is only obtained, as expected, if treatment begins when the colonies that are developing in the disc are near their maximum size. In this study, strains AL and GAD reached their maximum 10^7 bacteria/disc in 2 days and then stabilized, decreasing only 5 to 10 fold in 20 days. However, GAN grew slowly *in vivo;* after 8 days the number was not constant and sometimes suddenly dropped. In order to obtain the same inoculum strain, was cultivated first *in vivo* until the number per disc reached 10^7 to 10^8 bacteria per disc. Prior growth *in vivo* of small colonies does not modify the result *in vivo* as shown in a previous study.

Results

Minimum Inhibitory Concentrations of Strains

With an inoculum of 1×10^3 bacteria/spot, the following MIC's have been observed:

	Penicillin G U/ml	Streptomycin µg/ml
Streptococcus group D AL	2.5	100
Streptococcus group N GAN	0.5	16
Streptococcus group N GAD	0.5	16

The thiol-requiring strain GAD does not differ from Streptococcus group N—GAN.

By inoculating 10-fold dilutions from a suspension containing 10^7 bacterial/ml, strain GAD appeared to be twice as sensitive to penicillin as strain GAN when

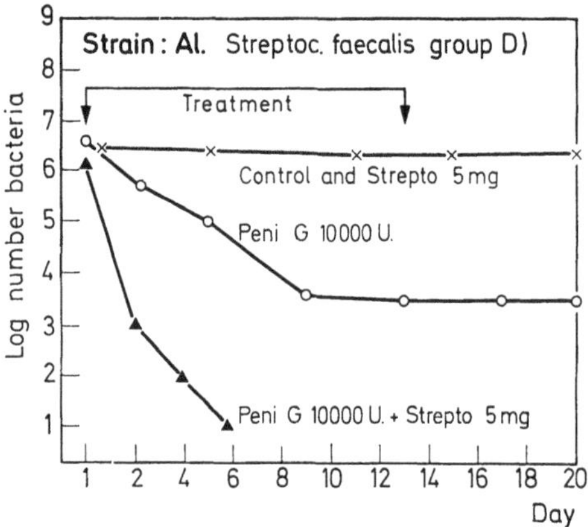

Fig. 1. Survivors of strain AL (*Str. faecalis* group D) in agar discs in the peritoneal cavity of mice

inocula of 1×10^2 to 1×10^3 bacteria/spot were used. Conversely, with a smaller inoculum, strain GAN appears to be twice as sensitive as strain GAD. Such differences are not sufficient to consider strain GAD as resistant.

Bactericidal Activity of Penicillin and Streptomycin in the Peritoneal Cavity of Mice

Streptococcus Group D—Strain AL

The results reported here, obtained with the same strain as studied previously, were almost the same (Fig. 3). The number of bacteria, 5×10^6 per disc, did not change in controls without treatment. Streptomycin (5 mg twice a day for 14 days) had no effect. Penicillin alone (1,000 U twice a day for 14 days) reduced the count to approximately 5×10^3 per disc in 9 days, and this number did not change until the end of the treatment (13 days). Ten days later, after stopping penicillin, the number of surviving bacteria was stable. These bacteria were in a persisting state because after cultivation *in vitro* they showed the same growth characteristics and the same MIC's as the initial population. It is difficult to establish how long the persistent state would continue without treatment. After 25 days, large discrepancies in the count of living bacteria were observed in different mice, or even between the two discs inserted in the peritoneal cavity of the same mouse. The phenomenon occurring at that time needs further studies.

The combination of both drugs was able to kill the inoculum in 6 days. This effect was much better than the effect of each antibiotic alone. Complete killing occurred more slowly in this experimental system than in the *in vitro* experiments.

Streptococcus Group N, Strain GAN

This strain was inhibited *in vitro* by lower inhibiting concentrations of streptomycin than the previous Streptococcus group D strain AL. Despite this, strepto-

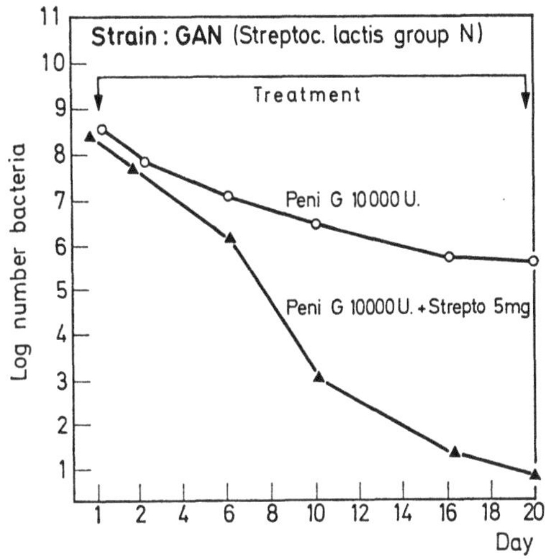

Fig. 2. Survivors of strain GAN (*Str. lactis* group N) in agar discs in the peritoneal cavity of mice

mycin 5 mg twice a day did not reduce the count of bacteria per disc *in vivo*. Penicillin G (10,000 U twice a day) reduced the count per disc from 1×10^8 bacteria per disc to around 10^5 bacteria per disc in 15 days. Although mice were treated for 20 days, the number of bacteria did not change significantly between the 15th and the 20th day of treatment. Approximately 10^5 bacteria/disc persisted (Fig. 2).

As mentioned under "Methods", this strain grows slowly *in vivo* in this experimental model, and large discrepancies in the counts of bacteria per disc were observed without treatment. In order to obtain a sufficient and stable number of control colonies, discs were incubated *in vitro* until the number of bacteria reached 1×10^8 bacteria/disc before they were inserted in the peritoneal cavity of mice. This inoculum, at the start of treatment, might be considered as different from the inoculum used for Streptococcus group D strain AL cultivated *in vivo* and treated when the bacterial count reached its maximum of 1×10^7 bacteria/disc.

In despite of this difference, the bacterial persistence state was established under treatment with penicillin G for both strains. This means (as shown in preliminary experiments) that it is important to start treatment when the colonial population reaches its maximum if one is to obtain a bacterial persistence phenomenon in this model. The fact that the peak count of the population has been obtained *in vitro* or *in vivo* is of minor importance, although, depending on the strains, this peak might be different *in vitro* and *in vivo*.

The combination of penicillin G and streptomycin killed the bacteria faster than each antibiotic separately. After 10 days of treatment, 1,000 times more survivors were observed with penicillin G alone than with the combination. Complete killing was obtained in this experiment between the 16th and 20th day of treatment.

Streptococcus Group N Thiol-Requiring Strain GAD

This deficient mutant is inhibited *in vitro* by the same concentration of penicillin and streptomycin as strain GAN. Streptomycin alone had no effect *in vivo*

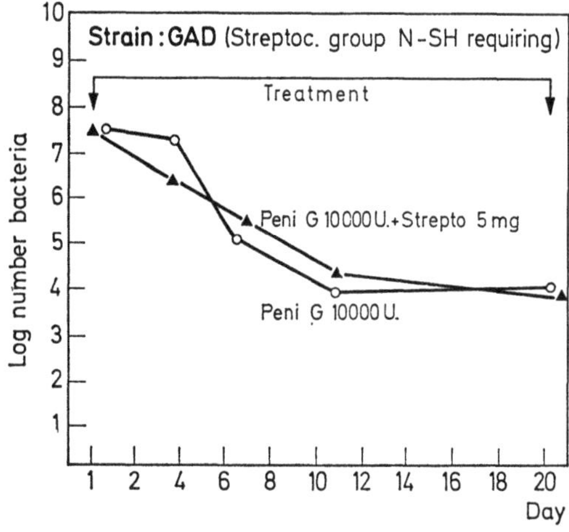

Fig. 3. Survivors of strain GAD (*Str.* group N SH-requiring) in agar discs in the peritoneal cavity of mice

on the count of bacteria per disc. Penicillin G alone reduced the count per disc from 3×10^7 bacteria/disc to around 1×10^4 bacteria/disc in 10 days and this number did not change until the treatment was stopped 10 days later. As with the previous strain, a state of bacterial persistence was observed in this experimental model with this deficient strain. The time needed for establishing this persistent state and the level of persisters was not much different from that required for the other strains (Fig. 3).

The only difference we observed was the effect of the penicillin-streptomycin combination. In contrast to the effect of this combination on the other strain, absolutely no synergistic effect occurred with the combination. In Fig. 3, the curve of decrease in the number of persisters obtained with the combination is exactly the same as shown in the curve obtained with penicillin alone. This lack of activity of the streptomycin in the combination is not related to a modification on the bacteriostatic activity of the streptomycin on the strain, the MIC being 16 µg/ml, as in the case of Streptococcus group N strain GAN.

Discussion

We developed an experimental model by inserting agar discs containing a small number of bacteria into the peritoneal cavity of mice. We then started treatment with penicillin G, streptomycin and their combination when colonies were fully grown. Counting of viable forming colony unit was performed during and after treatment. With streptococci of group D and group N, isolated by blood culture from untreated patients with bacterial endocarditis, we observed the following effects: streptomycin was not active. Penicillin G alone reduced the count slowly for about 10 days but further counting showed no change in the number of survivors. This occurred during treatment and after treatment was stopped during 20 days of observation. It can be assumed that bacterial persistence was obtained in this experimental model. The bacteria isolated after counting had the same growth characteristics and MIC's as the original strain. Their persistence may be considered as related to a phenotypic variation.

Penicillin G plus streptomycin in combination completely killed the inoculum or reduced it to less than ten bacteria in 6 to 15 days. As expected, this synergistic effect reproduced the phenomenon described by JAWETZ and GUNNISON 20 years ago. Conversely Streptococcus group N, isolated from an aortic valve after treatment by CAYEUX et al. and shown to be a deficient thiol-requiring mutant behaved differently when the mice were treated with the penicillin-streptomycin combination. This combination was no longer synergistic and bacterial persistence occurred just the same as with penicillin G treatment alone. Streptomycin had no effect on this type of organism despite the fact that the bacteriostatic MIC of streptomycin did not change.

This means that the drug and the environment in patients are able to select drug-sensitive bacteria with a genotypic variation. This mutant can persist under conditions where "normal" bacteria are killed.

Streptococcus group N strain GAD was not the only deficient strain with thiol-requirements isolated. Three additional strains with the same requirements have been isolated by CAYEUX et al.—two from a blood culture and one from a valve removed by cardiac surgery.

In these cases it might be said that one may only suspect that such strains are deficient thiol-requiring streptococci related to the Streptococcus initially infecting the patient.

Thiol-requiring deficient streptococci are not the only genotypic variants responsible for bacterial persistence. Other deficient streptococci have been isolated.

For instance, many years ago a patient with Streptococcus group D endocarditis, treated 4 days with a penicillin-streptomycin combination, developed allergy. After stopping treatment we isolated a slowly growing drug-sensitive

Streptococcus group D. It was able to back-mutate to the initial from. The speed of the bactericidal effect of antibiotics was slower for the deficient mutant.

On the other hand, it is common to isolate, mainly from chronic osteomyelitis slow-growing deficient staphylococci called G colonies by WISE et al. Many other examples of bacteria "deficient" as compared to "normal" forms have been reported in the literature and we do not intend to review this problem.

In conclusion, deficient drug sensitive variants may be selected *in vivo* by drugs or environment, in both treated and untreated patients. These variants persist *in vivo* and behave as bacteria of low pathogenicity. We also think that such bacteria are inadequately described merely by morphological or growth characteristics. A classification is only possible on the basis of their biochemical defect as we attempted to do with thiol-requiring streptococci.

References

CAYEUX, PH., ACAR, J. F., CHABBERT, Y. A.: Bacterial persistence in streptococcal endocarditis due to thiol requiring mutants. J. Infect. Dis., **124**, 241—254 (1971).

CHABBERT, Y. A., SUREAU, B., MARTIN, L. R., VIAL H.: Mécanisme d'action des antibiotiques dans les endocardites bactériennes a streptocoques. Memor. del IV Congreso Mundial de Cardiol. IV-B, 480—490 (1962).

GUZE, L. B. (Ed.): Microbial protoplasts, spheroplasts and L-forms. Baltimore: Williams and Wilkins Co. 1968.

JAWETZ, E., GUNNISON, J. B., COLEMAN, V. R.: Science **111**, 254 (1950).

LOURIA, D. B., KAMINSKI, T., GRIECO, H., SINGER, J.: Aberrant forms of bacteria and fungi found in blood or cerebrospinal fluid. Arch. intern. Med. **124**, 39—48 (1969).

McDERMOTT, W.: Microbial persistence. Yale J. Biol. Med. **30**, 257—291 (1958).

WAHL, R., CAYEUX, Ph.: Le clinicien devant les infections streptococciques. Maroc. méd. **45**, 497—500 (1966).

WERNER, C. A., KNIGHT, V., McDERMOTT, V.: Studies of microbial population artificially localized in vivo. I. Multiplication of bacteria and distribution of drug in agar loci. J. Clin. Invest. **33**, 742—752 (1954).

WISE, R. I., SPINK, W. W.: The influence of antibiotics on the origin of small (G variants) of *M. pyogenes var. aureus* J. Clin. Invest. **33**, 1611 (1954).

Dr. Y.-A. CHABBERT
Chef de Service Institut Pasteur
Bacteriologie Médicate
25 Rue du Docteur Roux
F-75 Paris XVᵉ

Discussion

KASS: Of course, the tremendous problem that we have to face is just when we should be looking for wall-deficient forms in the course of clinical disease. So far two, or possibly three models have shown up that suggest possibilities, — one in the urine, another in endocarditis, and perhaps a third in osteomyelitis. In the urine, so far, the evidence is that if wall-deficient forms account for chronicity, they must do so only rarely, because the only times wall-deficient forms have been isolated have been during or shortly after treatment. The majority of recurrent urinary infections we know to be due to reinfection with different strains; that could immediately remove the L-form from consideration. So it is only in the 10 or 15% that are due to the persistence of the same organism that wall deficient forms could account for chronicity in pyelonephritis. Many of us have looked very hard for L-forms in untreated chronic pyelonephritis, without success.

DASCHNER: As far as the relationship of antimicrobial treatment and the isolation of L-forms from urinary tract infections is concerned, GUTMAN [J. clin. Invest. 44, 1945 (1965)] described 11 patients with positive isolation of L-forms: 4 of these patients received no antimicrobial therapy at the time culture for bacterial variants was positive.

KASS: There have been problems in repeating these observations.

CHABBERT: I think that to be able to persist, such kind of bacteria have to be found in a quiet place. Perhaps the urinary tract is not a quiet place. I mean, for instance, the lesion of bacterial endocarditis is apparently a quiet place because colonies are surrounded by a sort of clot of fibrin. About coagulase-negative staphylococci in ventriculum shunts, I think that these forms may persist because they are not aggressive against the host. Also they are able to stay and perhaps to divide very slowly. The problem of reversion of defective forms probably depends on the size of the deletion in the chromosome. Bacteria with large deletions cannot revert, but they might induce some pathological effect, for instance, the defect in the heart valves.

HOLT: We are aware of this possibility; some years ago at Carlshalton, Prof. STEWART and I examined the contents of the shunt lumens for L-forms by the methods then available. We could demonstrate no L-forms, but what seem to be perfectly normal cocci.

FINLAND: In bacterial endocarditis it is not uncommon to find patients who come back many months after they were apparently cured, and if they come to autopsy, you sometimes grind up the valve and, with normal methods and media, cultivate the original organism. Some organisms must have persisted without change, at least with respect to growth in the medium that we used for culturing them. As a matter of fact, in the first experiences that we reported on the use of penicillin in endocarditis, we had several lapses. One was of particulai interest: the patient had an aortic insufficiency with a marked defect in the valve and positive blood cultures for several days before we started treatment. He was apparently cured, but he came back some months later with congestive heart failure and died. When we ground up the scarred, and apparently healed valve and sectioned it very carefully, no organisms were found in the sections. But interestingly enough, this patient had a large splenic abscess from which organisms, culturally identical with the original one that we had isolated from the blood, were grown in ordinary media.

We have other examples of patients to whom treatment has been given, for example, for a streptococcus, and we no longer can find that organisms, but after some time in the hospital they developed staphylococcol infections and died with staphylococcal endocarditis, and, when was cultured the valve at autopsy, we could still grow out the original Streptococcus as well as the Straphylococcus.

KASS: I would like to answer Dr. CHABBERT because this is a fascinating question and we must understand it. Since he has thought about this a great deal from the theoretical side, I would like to see if he can draw any more theoretical possibilities. Why does penicillin cure endocarditis? We say it is because it interferes with cell wall synthesis and any resulting protoplasts escape and undergo osmotic lysis in the isosmotic environment of the blood or tissues. We argue that wall-deficient forms cannot survive in the ordinary isosmotic environment of the body, otherwise penicillin would not be a useful drug. Now why should an L-form persist and not be killed under these conditions? We may have to postulate the occurrence of L-form mutants that are usually osmotically resistant or find circumstances of high osmotic activity such as we see in the renal medulla.

CHABBERT: L-forms have never been defined in terms of biochemical defect of the cell wall exactly, and it is clear, from the lecture by DASCHNER, that the requirement for sera are quite different from the ones you are speaking about. Stable-L-form types may result from a different mutation in the cell wall, and cell wall mutants are not the only defective mutants to be observed.

KASS: We could then argue that protoplasts are not synonymous.

DASCHNER: By no means. There is a great difference between L-forms and protoplasts. As I indicated, protoplasts are defined by the fact that they do not have any cell wall. HOFSCHNEIDER and MARTIN described *Proteus mirabilis* L-forms without any cell wall, or with a minimal cell wall structure. Different results in the literature may thus be explained by differences of the L-form itself, especially of the varying amount of cell wall material.

KASS: To what degree is it known whether the forms with different amounts of cell wall material are equally susceptible to osmotic lysis?

DASCHNER: I do not know of any study which has proved this.

BARTMANN: What Dr. DASCHNER has shown is the development of spheroplasts and the reversion of spheroplasts. You have also seen the survival of these large spheroplasts is limited, as is true also *in vitro*. If you observe the development of an L-form colony *in vitro* you can see that the propagation takes place in the agar by a process like budding. If these small cells come out of the agar they are enlarged and pushed away by other cells growing up from the depth, the so-called large bodies from the edge of the colony, and division of these large bodies is limited. After a certain period of time they are unable to divide and revert. I think if you try to explain a chronic infection or the occurrence of an infection *in vivo*, you should be able to demonstrate true propagation of the L-form instead of development, division and reversion under these conditions of large bodies *in vivo*. Have you seen anything like that?

DASCHNER: It has often been described that protoplasts and spheroplasts are not able to multiply. We were able to show that the bacterium as spheroplast is able to resume the ability to divide after inhibition by penicillin. If we inoculated these in urine-induced spheroplasts on salt-serum agar, most of the spheroplasts died or did not multiply. Some of them reverted to regular colonies of *Proteus mirabilis* and some of them grew as typical L-form colonies. As a matter of fact, the first slide I showed you (Fig. 1, p. 174) was an L-form colony obtained from urine-induced spheroplasts. These unstable L-form colonies reverted then over a period of 1 to 2 days to normal bacterial colonies.

BARTMANN: Have you any indication that these spheroplasts are able to survive for days and then revert ?

DASCHNER: In urine, no.

BARTMANN: I think this is important.

DASCHNER: Yes, Dr. BRAUDE showed that stable L-forms of *Proteus vulgaris* survived up to 1 week in rat kidney. KALMANSON and co-workers described a model where they demonstrated that streptococcus faecalis protoplasts were able to survive up to 13 weeks in rat kidney tissue.

VON GRAEVENITZ: I would like to ask Dr. DASCHNER what was the actual percentage of colony forming cells ?

DASCHNER: We have not yet performed such a quantitative study.

KASS: I would like to say, in relation to Prof. BARTMANN's important point, that in a kidney model with experimental enterococcal and staphylococcal infection where protoplasts had been demonstrated, there was persistence for many days in some of these, so it is at least theoretically possible.

FINLAND: I would like to recall that when Dr. THOMAS F. PAINE was working in my laboratory, the studies we made at that time were on the development of streptomycin-resistant and streptomycin-dependent forms and their reversion during cultivation from dependent to resistant and to normal forms. When we submitted the paper for publication, we had a group of photomicrographs of all the various forms that have been described of cell spheroplasts, of the elongated forms, filterable forms. The editor said that this was a well-known phenomenon and he would not publish the pictures, but he published the descriptions.[1]

Another observation we made at that time was in a patient with meningitis that followed surgery for brain abscess the original cultures were pure cultures of *Sreptococcus viridans*, but in doing repeated smears and cultures of the cerobrospinal fluid, Dr. PAINE saw some very bizarre forms and cultured the spinal fluid repeatedly on PPLO agar. He was thus able to demonstrate PPLO forms in the spinal fluid for a long period. During this time the patient seemed to improve, and eventually recovered completely, without demonstrating of any reversion to vegetative form. This was published in the Annals of Internal Medicine, 32, 554 (1950).

---

[1] PAINE, T. F., JR., FINLAND, M.: Observations on bacteria sensitive to, resistant to, and dependent upon streptomycin. J. Bact. **56**, 207—218 (1948).

Bayer-Symposium III, 201—204 (1971)

Epidemiological Investigations of R-Factor Bearing Enterobacteriaceae in Man and Animals in Germany

H. KNOTHE

With 1 Figure

In considering the addition of antibiotics to the feed of farm animals, two main questions are of great concern. 1. Do the low concentrations of antibiotics, usually mixed into the feed, exert a selective pressure sufficient to exert a wide

Table 1. *Occurence of resistant Enterobacteriaccae in the intestinal flora in three groups of individuals (in %)*

Resistance (Antibiotic)[a]	Healthy persons		Farm workers		Farm animals	
	total	R+	total	R+	total	R+
A	28	10	36	14	79	45
C	23	19	28	19	58	55
K	22	4	31	6	90	45
S	52	16	34	16	90	82
T	80	46	79	40	100	79

[a] A, ampicillin; C, chloramphenicol; K, kanamycin; S, streptomycin; T, tetracycline

selection of resistant organisms among Enterobacteriaceae ? 2. Does the increasing occurrence of resistant strains in such animals and in their environment profoundly influence the epidemiological situation in man, that is, can the resistant strains, emerging in animals, really cause infections or even epidemics in man which are difficult to manage with antibiotic treatment ?

The first question, namely, the overall origin of resistant bacteria under current feeding practices (in Germany 20 to 80 ppm) cannot be answered exactly at present because we cannot discriminate between the effect of antibiotic therapy from those of prophylaxis widely used on animal forms. However, it is a known fact that the proportion of resistant strains in and around farm animals is at present extremely high.

In the following, we intend to contribute to the elucidation of the second problem, namely the mutual relations of resistant strains found in man and animals with particular emphasis on strains with transferable resistance. The result of several series of epidemiological investigations performed by our group in Germany, in recent years, may throw some light on the situation.

Table 1 shows the percentage of strains from faeces of two groups of healthy persons and of animals. There was no significant difference in the incidence of resistance to individual antibiotics between healthy persons from a city population and those in daily contact with farm animals. However, animals from farms with intensive antibiotic feeding showed a marked increase in resistance to all antibiotics tested, with a particularly high incidence of R-factors.

If we consider the proportion of resistant cells in the total faecal enterobacterial flora (Table 2) we can see a shift from low incidence in healthy persons to an increased frequency of resistant bacteria in feces of farm workers, and even more in farm animals. The prevalence of a markedly resistant fecal flora in the last group and the total absence of stools with sensitive bacteria, must be interpreted as being caused by continous and long-term use of antibiotics in feed, as well as in prophylaxis and treatment of the animals.

The prevalence of R-factor-bearing strains and their distribution in feces of various groups of persons and farm animals—which might be regarded as repre-

Table 2. *Quantitative proportion of resistant cells among the total enterobacterial flora in three groups of individuals (in %)*

Source		Less than 10^{-2} %	10^{-4}—10^{-2} %	10^{-2}—1 %	over 1 %
Healthy	total	27	34	32	1
Persons	R^+	8	16	14	7
Farm	total	7	25	34	33
Workers	R^+	3	9	12	12
Farm	total	—	3	27	70
Animals	R^+	—	2	14	31

sentative for Germany—is given in Fig. 1. Again resistant organisms in the fecal flora are present in all animals examined and in different proportions compared to the number of susceptible cells. In various groups of healthy persons the situation seems to be more favourable at present with regard to the presence of R-factors. We divided the persons connected with animals into three groups:

1. Farm workers directly in contact with animals.

2. Their relatives who have no direct contact with either animals or animal feed, and

3. the feeding staff, i.e. persons handling only the animal feed and thus coming into close contact with antibiotic substances and less with bacterial strains.

In the last group, most of the resistance observed seems to be chromosomal, in contrast to that caused by R-factors which is prevalent in the first two groups. In Fig. 1, the two remaining groups of persons (city population and slaughterhouse workers) were not in contact with antibiotics, but the latter group may be exposed to resistant strains during professional handling of animals.

Table 3 shows the incidence of resistance among strains of *Salmonella typhimuirum* in Germany and the proportion of strains with transferable resistance. Altogether 136 resistant strains of human origin and 524 resistant strains of animal origin were investigated for resistance transfer. We found that as much as

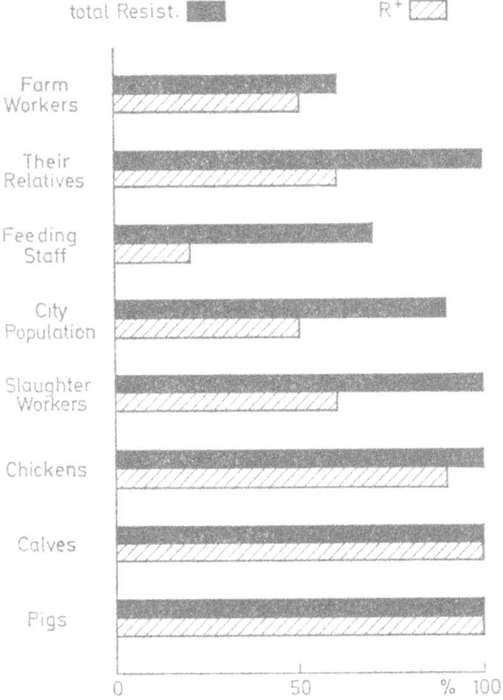

Fig. 1. Percentage of individuals with resistant Enterobacteriaceae

Table 3. *Incidence of resistant S. typhimurium in persons and animals in Germany (in %)*

	A	C	K	S	T
Persons (n = 136)					
total	13	6	1	29	45
R+	12	4	1	7	41
Animals (n = 524)					
total	43	0,5	3	28	55
R+	40	0,5	3	11	49

90% of ampicillin and tetracycline-resistance is transferable in both human and animal strains of *Salmonella typhimurium*. We were also able to isolate as many as six strains with transferable chlorampenicol-resistance. This disturbing fact supports the recommendation of the Swann report for restriction of chloramphenicol in most human usage.

The incidence of tetracycline-resistance, and, in animals, of ampicillin-resistance, as well, remains at a constantly high level in Germany from our data in 1967. We may assume that strains of Salmonella from man are most frequently isolated before therapy is started but that in animals, the sampling of feces and isolation of strains is usually accomplished during therapy. Therefore, one is justified in regarding the figures of animal strains in Table 3 with some caution.

The data we presented dealt with only a few aspects of the epidemiological significance of transferable resistance in Germany. Nevertheless, they strongly point to the growing importance of an overall unfavourable situation: the gradual loss of antibiotic susceptibility of enterobacterial strains currently seen.

Prof. Dr. H. KNOTHE
Direktor des Hygiene-Instituts
der Universität Frankfurt
D-6000 Frankfurt (Main)
Paul-Ehrlich-Straße 40

Discussion

FINLAND: Is there anybody here who is well acquainted with the SWANN report who might tell us about some of its repercussions. Prof. SHOOTER and Prof. WILLIAMS were either of you on the commission? (No) That is good, then you can give us an unbiased account, or perhaps an account tainted with your own bias.

SHOOTER: In my view we are very short of facts in this field and our quarrel, as a group, with the SWANN report was that it suggested that animal strains of *E. coli* might, and could, reach humans but would not establish themselves. In our view they do establish themselves and if this is the case this paper is an interesting forecast of damage that might come in the future.

FINLAND: Is it clearly established that disease in humans due to these forms are traceable to these animals?

SHOOTER: We have had strains which we have found in food and in the patients' stool which subsequently caused infections of the same type. We have had the same strains in the slaughter house meat, in food, and in patients' stools, but in the study they did *not* produce sepsis as well. I have little doubt that the strains which our patients are taking in are establishing themselves in the bowel, and that some of these are the ones that turn up in the urinary tract.

FINLAND: How do you know that they did not come from those that handled the food before it was delivered to the patients?

SHOOTER: This is an obvious possibility. We have tried to get round it by taking swabs of cows and chickens just before and immediately after they were killed; during the process of flaying the carcass. In the course of cutting up the meat strains, spread from one animal to another. We have had the same meat delivered to us and it arrives in the hospital with the strains that we found before. They may have been added by people on the way but they are still of the same types as the ones we had originally.

I do not want to overdo this but I think this is one route by which infection comes and new strains arrive.

Pulverer: Normally the strains of staphylococci in animals and humans are quite different but you can clearly find human strains in animal infections and bovine strains in human infections. This is possible.

von Graevenitz: I would assume that A.C.K.S.T. stand for ampicillin, chloramphenicol, kanamycin, streptomycin and tetracycline.

Shooter: Yes.

Ericsson: To my mind the main problem is whether bacteria from animals are capable of entering the human body and cause disease. Some years ago we had in Sweden the biggest outbreak of *Salmonella breslau* ever observed; 10,000 cases were notified and perhaps 5 to 7 times more are estimated to have occurred. There is no doubt that the epidemic emanated from infected animals. Apart from general biological consideration of the risk of creating pools of resistance factors, this is the main reason for the restrictive attitude taken by the medical profession, veterinarians and administrators to the use of antibiotics in animal feeds. The basic idea is that no substance which might be considered for use in humans should ever be used for growth promotion in animals.

Finland: I would like to ask one question. Why is it that, in an outbreak of Salmonella infection, whether due to animals, chickens or food handlers, it necessarily has anything to do with the feeding of antibiotics to animals? That is the real question. In our experience these organisms (i.e. Salmonella) are susceptible to antibiotics by the time that we get them and, moreover, even though they are susceptible in vitro, the infections do not respond to antibiotics; that is true of Salmonella as a group. So what is the problem here?

Antibiotics have been used for animal feeding now in the United States for something like 20 years and in most other countries for 15 years and the R-factor has been discussed for the last 5 or 6 years. Yet, as far as anybody can tell, the number of animal bacteria transferred to humans has not suddenly exploded into large epedemic over last 20 years. The time when it certainly should have exploded was within the first couple of years where, in every feed lot, it was shown that after feeding for a very short time you get a predominance of resistant strains.

Ericsson: My question is whether, in the long run, antibiotics has any growth promoting effect when given in animal food?

Finland: The antibiotics make money for the producers that is why they use them, otherwise they would not. The point is they use them only in two situations. They use them in the way we do to *treat* infection. Some of them use antibiotics, as some doctors do in hospitals, for prophylaxis of infections. But a great majority of them use them during the early weeks of life because it has been shown empirically that there is a heavier animal at the end of the first few weeks, and this is worth millions of dollars to a producer. They *stop* feeding antibiotics after this time. This raises one problem. The other time when antibiotics are used is at the time of slaughter, the idea being that they feed these animals intensively in crowded "feed lots", and they may transfer many bacteria, some of which, under the conditions of feeding, may be pathogenic. They want to reduce the amount of bacterial content of the carcass, and it also increases the shelf-life of the meat. Now this latter use raises the problem of antibiotics residue which might have been transferred to humans and therefore raises problems of sensitization or development of a resistant infection. The most important use of antibiotics, for which the greatest proportion of antibiotics are used, however, is in the early weeks to increase body weight.

ERICSSON: Prof. FINLAND, I am quite aware of all the facts which you have presented but I thoroughly disagree with your conclusions and recommendations. I do not think there there is good scientific evidence for the growth promoting effect of antibiotics in the long run, I think that the tests carried out have been run during periods that are too short and have only registered the first favourable effect on stable hygiene, just as we have in the hospital observed a temporary effect on prophylactic use of antibiotics. There is also a bad practice amongst farmers that sick animals are given extra antibiotics in order to cover the disease for the veterinarians of a slaughter house. If antibiotics are given in the same situation to increase the shelf-life of the meat, this is certainly another example of bad practice.

FINLAND: Well, I think that if the increase in weight of animals is not something which the great animal food industry thinks is statistically significant, they would long since have stopped using antibiotics. They have studied this pretty extensively. The problem has been studied in experimental stations in several universities in the United States and Canada and in Europe, and the data are all there. I suppose one can interpret the data one way or another but apparently the animal farmers, the animal food producers think they are making money, otherwise they would not spend it for this purpose.

KASS: May I ask a question about Dr. KNOTHE's paper. I do not know whether Dr. VON GRAEVENITZ can answer it but perhaps he could transmit this for the proceedings of the discussion. I am assuming, as did Prof. ERICSSON, that what happened here is that the specimens were spread on plates containing antibiotics and that what is reported fundamentally is "any" resistance. The difficulty with that is, of course, that we have no controls left because this method is not quantitative and we do not know with what to compare it. Looking over these data, one sees, for example, that the feeding staff is better off than the city population. Now this could be interpreted that the galloping epidemic of resistant organisms which first spread from the farm to the city, now has spread back to the farm. But it could also be interpreted as none of these, only this method is so unquantitative that, on the random basis, we are picking up some extra resistant organism which has come out this way. One would like to know what the city population, or the people working around the hospital, for example, are likely to pick up at random in the form of resistant strains and if this would be very much higher than, let us say, among the people working out on the edge of the city. I am afraid that for me, these data cannot be interpreted. I would like to hear some interpretations before any conclusions are drawn, one way or the other, about animal feed, antibiotics or anything else.

FINLAND: I think that Dr. VON GRAEVENITZ can be excused from answering any of these questions but I would hope that Prof. BARTMANN or one of his associates here would convey all of these questions to Dr. KNOTHE so that when this discussion actually appears in the publication, these questions will be answered.

SHOOTER: I should like to ask Prof. KASS whether, in fact, he has any figures for the enteric bacteria of either poultry, cows or pigs in the United States just before slaughter, which is the operative time?

KASS: No, I just do not follow these data as closely as I should. I think I should get into it, based upon this discussion and look more closely at it. I hope, however, that no one will trust data that are non-quantitative or any data that are obtained simply by streaking on plates containing concentration of antibiotic that simply uncover an unstable percentage of the total flora. This cannot be useful to us. This must be done by the very difficult method of total quantitation and the percentage or resistant strains in relation to this total. I do not think many people have done this because it involves a tremendous amount of work. To give you an example, one of our house officers, a pharmacologist, had amebiasis. During his elective time with us, he wanted to take tetracycline and we convinced him that he should do serial counts of his fecal flora before, during, and then just after the treatment, to get some idea of the changes that would occur. Well, it took this man a whole month to get this series of cultures done on himself! This is the way it is and anyone who has worked with stool bacteriology knows exactly what I mean. This is a difficult thing to do properly. But I would stress that unless it is done properly, we would not be able to interpret the data.

SHOOTER: Yes.

FINLAND: There have now been several conferences on this subject, one was at the National Academy of Science in Washington in the middle 50's and reported in a monograph published by the Academy. Another one was held in Washington 2 years ago and the results of that conference have also been published. There was also a recent one again in England and, I presume, it has been, or will be, published. I think that they all produced the same inconclusive results, with some people arguing vigorously for the elimination of antibiotics in animal feeds. Others say that when you show us why, then you will have an argument, but you have not shown us why, because there are equal arguments to the contrary. I do not think we shall answer that question unless it is shown that some disease is regularly produced in humans by this transfer of resistant organisms from animals to the patients and that we cannot treat them adequately bacause the organisms are resistant to antibiotics by virtue of the animals having been subjected to the antibiotics in their feed.

The fact unfortunately is that the population is increasing and we have not reduced the population by the feeding of antibiotics to animals.

VON GRAEVENITZ: I do have a question to Dr. KNOTHE, namely, how high is the percentage of resistant enterobacteria after the animals have *not* received feed with antibiotics for, say, 2 years, and also: how is the percentage of resistant enterobacteria in farmworkers 2 years after they have changed their profession?

Bayer-Symposium III, 209—219 (1971)
© by Springer-Verlag 1971

General Discussion

GOULD: In making some general remarks I would like to suggest that we do not go on record as making the mistake of forming an anti-antibiotic crusade. There seems to be a tendency when microbiologists interested in antibiotics get together, to give the impression of exaggerating the harmful effects of these agents, particularly with respect to antibiotic-resistant strains. Prof. WILLIAMS, earlier today, did hint at this when he referred back to the literature about staphylococci in the early and mid 1950's. If one goes back and looks at this literature one does indeed get the impression that antibiotic-resistant staphylococci were preponderant in infections. I think that this exaggerated reporting is showing itself again in our discussions on the transfer of resistance amongst micro-organisms (infectious resistance) and in the possible transfer of resistant pathogens from animals to man. There is no doubt that the mechanisms for the development of antibiotic-resistance in organisms, whether by transduction, transformation or conjugation followed by genetic transfer do occur and that selection of resistant genotypes can be encouraged by the use of antibiotics, but the important question is how much do they actually influence the population at large?

I consider it most important that this is not exaggerated. I would suggest on our own limited experience in the northern part of the United Kingdom that, at the present time, the influence is very small indeed and certainly the evidence for the transfer of antibiotic-resistant enterobacteriaceae from animals to man is very small. In relation to the gram-positive cocci such as Staphylococcus, anti-biotic-resistance is now a much lesser problem than it was 10 years ago. However, I would not suggest that there is no need for vigilance, but this should be one of the main functions of laboratories who maintain a monitoring activity in relation to determining the current antibiotic sensitivity of bacteria.

The same general remarks should be emphasised in relation to the isolation of basically resistant species which have frequently been referred to, and I, myself, discussed under the heading of "opportunists in infection". It must be emphasised that infections due to these organisms affect only a minority of patients although in some units the proportion affected may be somewhat larger, particularly when they are dealing with rather specialised types of patients which allows more ready selection for growth of these resistant bacteria.

I think it would be a very bad thing for us to lose sight of the fact that anti-biotics remain predominantly beneficial and useful in the control of infection in man and animals. It is an ideal to suggest that antibiotics should not be used prophylactically because many of our clinical colleagues are satisfied that patients benefit from such use; it is all very well to say that antibiotics should only be prescribed after we have established a diagnosis and determined the sensitivity of the organism to specific antibiotics, but in practice this is something which we simply cannot attain. Even in the most highly developed countries I would suggest that more than 90% of patients with clinical infection are treated with antibiotics without any bacteriological examination or attempt at selecting the antibiotic on the basis of specific laboratory tests. Fortunately for us as doctors the great majority of patients get better under these conditions and in relation to our present discussions we must ask, is there really such a drastic effect upon the bacterial population because of this policy?

My own opinion is that instead of attempting to insist upon greater control of individual antibiotics, that we examine in greater detail the effect of general policies in the use of antibiotics in the community and the way in which such controlled use modifies the general epidemiological pattern of resistant organisms.

WILLIAMS: I feel rather surprised that we have not talked about the longer term trends in the infective disease and the extent to which these can be explained on the basis of possible changes in the microorganisms. I showed, in my paper, the mortality from puerperal sepsis and I pointed out that in about 1935 the curve came down very sharply. Although in Britain the definition of "peurperal sepsis" has been changed several times, it appears that the mortality was rising in the second half of the last century. At the same time the other great killer among the streptococcal infections, scarlet fever, showed a decline in mortality, which in 1856 was of the order of 2,000/million children, down to about 20/million, long before there was any significant effect of antibiotics. In Britain and in the United States scarlet fever has been a very mild disease in the last 3 or 4 decades. Of course, the same thing could be shown for diphtheria, the mortality from this decreased long before the introduction of prophylactic immunisation. I wonder whether these long term changes in the incidence of the major classical infective diseases were due to changes in the micro-organisms, or whether they were due to changes in the social circumstances in which the population was living, or could it be that the changes in the social circumstances, were, in fact, inflicting a change upon the microorganisms.

I have often wondered whether the pattern of streptococcal infection in the United States Armed Forced in the 1940's reflects this fact that, if streptococci are given good opportunities for passing around in the human population rapidly and frequently, they achieve enhanced virulence. Perhaps if the role of spread is reduced, not only does this reduce the chances of an individual becoming infected but it also gradually attenuates the virulence of the organism. With streptococci this can be done in the laboratory; if you pass streptococci successively through mice you certainly will enhance their virulence. I wonder whether there are any other examples of a long term change in the virulence of some of the other micro-organisms which we have been talking about that could be regarded as analogous to the sort of picture which I claim we have seen with Streptococcus in the last century.

KASS: A critical problem, to me, is in this term virulence, which at the moment is being looked at from the point of view of the structure of the microorganism. If we broaden the definition, we may choose to look at the situation also from the point of view of size of inoculum. The studies in England on the spread of rheumatic fever in the 1920's showed a very strong correlation between frequency of rheumatic heart disease and numbers of people per room. This suggests that a factor in the improved health of recent years has been more dilute housing. One of the most telling examples of this has come from recent studies of LILIENFELD and his associates. In Baltimore, where rheumatic fever has continued to be seen, what was puzzling was that the Negro families with rheumatic fever were often middle class families on the basis of their incomes. Further studies of these families showed that there was no longer an adequate correlation between rate of rheumatic fever and income level or educational level but there was continued correlation with the number of people per bedroom. What had apparently happened was that as the family climbed out of the slums, and was buying a new house, a choice was often necessary between buying maximal space in the dining room or in the bedroom. It turned out that the bedroom space was more readily sacrificed and the crowding in the bedroom was maintained, so that, for 8 to 12 h the children had close association with one another. I am deeply concerned whether the critical factor is inoculum size fully as much as any biological changes in the organisms, because what we know about the known properties of the organisms indicates that these have not changed. I therefore find little evidence for a change in virulence of the organisms and would suggest that the inoculum size may be a more relevant variable to explain what we have seen.

GSELL: The long-term patterns of infectious disease show very well the different effects of the social hygienic conditions on the macro-organism and of chemotherapy on the micro-organisms. As Dr. WILLIAMS mentioned, for the last 40 years we could demonstrate this for the mortality of tuberculosis, of pneumonias and other infectious diseases [Antibiot. et Chemother. (Basel) 14, 1 (1968)]. I can demonstrate here the wonderful table of the Office of Health Economics in Great Britain for *pneumonia*, not only for the last years but for 100 years from 1860 to 1960 (Fig. 1). The mortality goes up until 1900 as a result of the industrial revolution, the slums and poor hygienic conditions and naturally also by the evolution of the population.

Then it goes down slowly till 1939, then precipitously after the introduction of sulfonamides and of antibiotics. The decrease can be shown during the following 15 years and the mortality of pneumonia stays now on a low level. The stop of the decrease is caused by the persisting high mortality for infants and for very old people; those over 75. In these two groups the condition of the macroorganism predominates and overshadows the possibilities of the action of antibiotics. In a second table of the American Life Insurance Company, from the age of 1 year to 74 years, that is, excluding infants and older age groups, we see the dramatic effect on pneumonia mortality of the sulfonamides, then a second decrease by penicillin and a third one by the introduction of Aureomycin. From 1949 to 1965, the mortality rate stayed on the low level but with the predominance of older people in our population, the mortality goes slowly up from 13,2 per 100,000 persons to 20,5 (1963) and 18,5 (1964) (Fig. 2).

In the *epidemiology of bacteremia* it is interesting that in the last 10 to 20 years, the number of bacteremias caused by microorganisms of low-pathogenity has risen. Not only the diseases due to gram-negative bacteria, as we can see it in the statistics given by Dr. FINLAND and Dr. KASS, but also those due to other *bacteria of low-pathogenity*, are seen *more often*. It is not due to the resistance to antibiotics

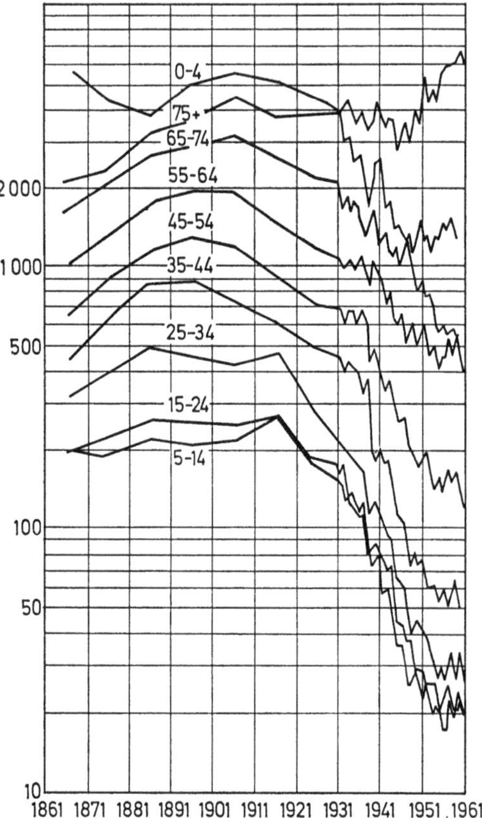

Fig. 1. Mortality from pneumonia in England and Wales from 1861—1961 (per million population) (from 1861—1930 the data for each 10 years, and from 1931—1961 the curve shows annual rates)

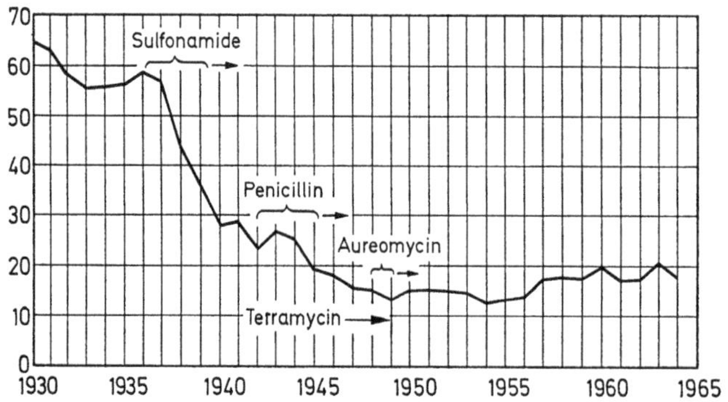

Fig. 2. Pneumonia mortality (per 100,000 population) (1 to 74 years of age). Effects of Sulfonamides and antibiotics, 1936 to 1965 (Amer. Life Ins. Co.)

because we now have other effective products against these micro-organisms but the general effect of newer treatments by chemotherapy for cancer and other diseases and by immuno-suppressive agents with toxic side-effects, especially on the bone-marrow. Now saprophytic bacteria can become pathogenic (p. 146). This has presented to the clinician and to the bacteriologist a new aspect of very dangerous illnesses.

ERICSSON: You asked me, Dr. FINLAND, about the general value of this conference. As at most conferences and especially the small ones, I think that the personal contact and the opportunity directly to exchange information with colleagues who are interested in the same problems, is most rewarding.

As to the general topic of our conference, the changing pattern of etiology of infections, I would, to some extent, dispute the opinion of Dr. KASS. There have certainly been changes for which the reasons are very obscure. The tendency to attribute the changes to preventive or therapeutic methods underestimates the unknown factors and the spontaneous changes. The reduction of diphtheria during the later part of the 19th and the beginning of the 20th century can certainly not be ascribed to specific therapy, and the reduction after the second world war can hardly be ascribed to prophylactic measures.

I also think, Dr. WILLIAMS, that if you are going to ascribe the reduction of puerperal fever in the U.K. to the introduction of sulfonamides, you must have started using this substance generally in your country before it was available in any other country.

I, myself, am inclined to believe more in the effect of antibiotics in small epidemiological units where the selective pressure of antibiotics may really exert all its effect. This is, in my opinion, mainly a negative effect, as the emergence of resistant strains, and the change of prevailing species within hospitals has not reduced the occurrence of hospital cross-infections or made their treatment any easier. Therefore, we have in the Karolinska Hospital been very concerned with the "rational use of antibiotics". This was the title of my academic thesis, it has become my "red herring" and I hope that it will be my last will!

FINLAND: So we have had a confirmation of your attitude. I am sure that everyone adheres to the same general principle with respect to antibiotics. We are here, and wherever we gather, for the purpose of learning the best way to use them for the benefit of our patients.

BARTMANN: I would like to pick up again this problem of socio-economic influences, especially after what Dr. KASS has said. We in Berlin are studying the infections in children caused by isoniazid-resistant tubercle bacillus, mainly the aspect concerned with changes in virulence, but we can leave this for the moment. We have also looked at the epidemiological background and one interesting thing turned up. We have followed the incidence, over the years and have seen that the number of children infected and having disease caused by tubercle bacilli became lower and lower. At the same time, the incidence in the adult population was rising. We have looked for the reasons for this. We have compared standardised groups infected by bacilli sensitive or resistant to antituberculous drugs. There was one main difference and this was the housing conditions. We then looked for the changes in these conditions and we could establish a correlation. The housing conditions became better and better. At the same time, BCG vaccination was introduced on a mass scale for the newborns.

REBER: The subject of this present symposium: "Bacterial infections: changes of their causative agents" can be considered under two aspects. The first concerns the changes in relation to time and locality which has been principally discussed in this symposium. The second aspect concerns the change of the bacterial flora during an infection in an individual patient, essentially under chemotherapy. We have studied this problem as related to the infections which occurred at the Basle University Medical Clinical in 1963. Out of 3,700 patients, 650 could be retained to estimate the effect of antibiotic treatment in infections. Limiting our investiga-

Table 1. *Change of the microbial flora in bronchitis and bronchopneumonia*

Result	Number of cases				
	Bronchitis		Bronchopneumonia		Total
	acute	chronic	acute	chronic	
Cured	34	32	35	8	109
Partially cured	—	2	—	2	4
Failures	12	12	7	4	35
Microbial change	11	17	4	4	36
Total	57	63	46	18	184
% changes in flora	19	27	8	22	

tions to the broncho-pulmonary and the urinary infection, we found the following results:

Among 120 cases of bronchitis, 28 presented a change of the original bacterial flora after a course of antibacterial treatment: among 64 cases of broncho-pneumonia, 8 showed a change (Table 1). Of 74 chronic cases with urinary tract infections, 27 (36%) presented a change of the bacterial flora under treatment and out of 76 acute or subacute cases (or acute exacerbations) 17 (22%). The difference between the acute and the chronic cases is statistically significant (Table 2).

In all these cases, we have not attempted to verify the causative role of the isolated microorganisms by serological reactions; in the urinary tract infections, only significant bacteriurias, following KASS' definition, were considered. So we prefer the expression "changes of the microbial flora" instead "change of causative agents".

Four factors must be considered:

— the terrain, on which the infection is developing,
— primary flora,
— the chemotherapy,
— the secondary flora.

Not every infection is followed by a change of microbial flora. In typhoid fever, for example, this phenomenon is not known. Perhaps it happens in the presence of an underlining disease which pre-disposes to a fixation of microorganisms. Anatomical or functional lesions of the superficial epithelial layer or diminutions of the cellular or humoral defence mechanisms are generally involved and con-

Table 2. *Change of the microbial flora in urinary infections*

Result	Chronic	Subacute	Acute remission	Acute	Total
Not conclusive	25	14	26	8	73
Cured	17	6	12	3	38
Partially cured	8	4	0	1	13
Failures	22	12	17	4	55
Microbial change	27	3	11	3	44
Total	74	25	40	11	150
% change in flora	36	12	27	27	

Table 3. *Change of the microbial flora in urinary infections (most frequent germs)*

Species	Initial organisms[a]			Second organisms[d]			No change[e]
	total	single[b]	mixed[c]	total	single	mixed	
E. coli	25	12	13	12	3	9	13
Str. faecalis	15	4	11	16	6	10	9
Proteus (vulgaris etc.)	9	3	6	16	3	13	8
Pseudomonas	3	1	2	1	—	1	1

Flora in urinary infections without change of the microbial flora[f]

E. coli	69	33	36
Str. faecalis	22	4	18
Proteus	27	7	20
Pseudomonas	8	1	7
Staph. aureus	5	2	3

[a] Bacterial species isolated at the beginning of the treatment.
[b] Monoinfection.
[c] Mixed infection.
[d] Bacterial species isolated after change of the microbial flora.
[e] Persistence of the initial species, addition of new species.
[f] Distribution of species in urinary infections without change of the microbial flora.

tinue to present favourable conditions for an infection even when a primary agent is eliminated by chemotherapy.

The species of the primary bacterial agent is not a predisposing factor for a change of the flora, except in certain virus diseases (influenza, etc.). Effective chemotherapy seems to be an essential condition for a microbial change. The nature of the antibiotic plays a role in the sense that a bactericidal substance with a wide spectrum limits the possibilities of a secondary infection by reducing the eligible bacteria.

The nature of the secondary invader depends on the circumstances, i.e. the presence of sources of infection and the extent of the chemotherapeutic barrier (Table 3). The secondary invader has the properties of resistance to the chemotherapy utilised and limited nutritional requirements.

The secondary invader is transmitted by autoinfaction or by cross-infection, essentially in the framework of hospital infection.

This was an attempt to see in a given hospital population, number of changes in organisms that occur under treatment.

FINLAND: I presume that by change you mean different bacteria, not just change of resistance in the same bacteria.

WYSOCKI: I think you will agree that there is some difference between the point of view of the microbiologists and that of the clinicians concerning antibacterial chemoprophylaxis, and I think you agree that there are some patients in whom antibacterial chemoprophylaxis is more advantageous than harmful.

For example, in operative procedures for mitral stenosis of rheumatic origin, or prophylaxis in severely injured patients in avoiding gas gangrene. My question addressed to the microbiologists is—could you tell me, from your point of view, in what kind of disease and in what kind of patient should we, as clinicians, be allowed to use antibacterial chemoprophylaxis?

FINLAND: Well, I do not know whether I can choose each end of the spectrum but I certainly can choose one end and I shall ask Dr. ERICSSON, before we go on to Dr. KASS, to give his point of view.

ERICSSON: I do admit that there are situations in which chemoprophylaxis is indicated. You probably mentioned the best one which is the prevention of relapse in rheumatic fever. I think that there is a general agreement on this point all over the world.

However, when you analyse other indications one after the other, you will find that they are very doubtful from the general biological point of view and that careful investigators have failed to show their effect. "Enterobiotic" has ,for instance, been shown to be a good laxative which may, however, lead to serious disturbances of the natural flora of the bowel. Nobody has conclusively shown that these changes reduce the risk of operations.

As to the care of the unconscious patient, another indication for routine prophylaxis, it has been shown by investigators in Seattle who treated every second patient, that the frequency of pulmonary complication is not reduced by prophylaxis. The complications were more severe in the treated group.

The main approach to antibiotic prophylaxis must be selective. We should know what we are aiming at and always prefer a rifle to a shot-gun.

Prof. BARTMANN, you questioned whether the microbiologist or the clinician should evaluate the result of chemoprophylaxis. I think that neither of them should do it alone. The effect should be evaluated in close collaboration between clinicians and clinical microbiologists. My thesis "rational use of antibiotics in hospitals" contains 27 references to papers from our hospital resulting from such collaboration. They all tend to illustrate problems I raised and points I made.

BARTMANN: I entirely agree.

FINLAND: Does anybody want to defend the use of prophylactic antibiotics, except under conditions where you are aiming at something that you clearly expect and specifically shoot for well-defined organisms with a specifically directed agent ?

BARTMANN: I would not like to defend, but I would like to reply to the question of Dr. WYSOCKI. I wonder whether the microbiologist is the right man to give you an answer. I think this has to be tested very carefully in controlled trials by the clinician, as just mentioned by Dr. ERICSSON.

FINLAND: My first summary about the prophylactic use of antibiotics was made before the New York Academy of Medicine a good many years ago [1] and at that time I indicated there were certain people who would give antibiotics to the mother before the baby was born, to the baby after it was born and they would find an excuse for giving antibiotics until the time they died and were interred. They would then inject antibiotics to make sure that deterioration of the body was slowed down or prevented. But continually reviewing the problem of prophylaxis, we find that every time a prophylactic agent has been introduced by somebody in prophylaxis for a specific purpose, it always worked very well until it was used for some time. Then, even under the same conditions, the effect of this prophylaxis disappeared very rapidly. In a recent discussion, a good academic surgeon advocated the prophylactic use in surgery of a drug cephaloridine, which some people had felt was a rather dangerous drug to use indiscriminately because of its tendency to produce renal disease. This was for prophylaxis during surgery, and we know that some patients develop lowblood pressure and they might develop defects in excretion and reduced renal function after that, and, therefore, it was not a very good antibiotic to use under such circumstances. He showed a controlled study in which he had practically no infections among the prophylactically treated cases and got the expected number in the untreated cases. When he was challenged by the panel and asked "do you use this prophylaxis in your surgical practice" ? he said "No", this was just a study. In the use of antibiotics for preparation of the bowel before colonic surgery, which is an obvious situation, those who have had careful bacteriological and antibiotic control have given this up. But there is one surgeon who has not given it up, and each year he uses a different antibiotic and always reports good results. However he has never published his mortality figures. When he was challenged at one time, he admitted that he had the same mortality rate, and infection rate, in his patients as anybody else who did not use prophylactic antibiotic preparation for surgery of the colon.

WYSOCKI: To answer the question of Prof. BARTMANN. I am sure that we, as clinicians, have to perform controlled trials to approach this problem.

KASS: Although it is generally agreed that prophylaxis of the patient with mitral disease before surgery is a good thing, no one has advanced proof that prophylaxis is effective. The idea is a projection from a reasonable view about the streptococcus and its relation to penicillin and from the knowledge that penicillin is a relatively harmless drug. However, a controlled trial that proves the effectiveness of prophylactic penicillin in patients with mitral disease does not exist.

We should be clear about what are facts and what are reasonable derivations from the facts and, of course, should try to determine what is pure fancy.

I raise these problems because of our discussion of the role of socioeconomic change in infections. In almost every western country in which there are data, as Prof. WILLIAMS outlined earlier, the decline in rates of certain communicable diseases has occurred independently of specific therapeutic or prophylactic intervention. For example, the decline in mortality from tuberculosis in England started from about 1850 and in the state of Massachusetts by about 1860. The decline was essentially linear until about 1955 and the curves show no place where the effect of the discovery of the tubercle bacillus, the effect of BGG, the effect of streptomycin, or of tuberculin testing influenced the rate of decline. The only things that influenced the rate of decline was wars. In all of these curves, the poor come off worse than the rich and the only time that the curve begins to change at all is after the discovery of isoniazid, and by then mortality from tuberculosis was but a tiny fraction of what is was in 1850. The same kind of trend is seen for diphtheria, scarlet fever, pertussis and measles, except that the downward trend starts about 20 years later than for tuberculosis. Again one cannot see from the curves where any specific interventions were instituted.

The reason for stressing these well-known points is that we still do not know what happened. These changes are the most important events in the history of the health of mankind, yet we are in the unhappy position that the mechanism is unexplained. We may speculate whether it is due to less crowding, or to improved nutrition, or to other factors, but we do not know.

It is also well established that there are other forms of infections (and this comes back to the point Prof. GSELL raised), such as poliomyelitis and perhaps infectious hepatitis, in which antibody immunity is the key to natural immunity and in this group of infections, the statistics get better. In the latter group, vaccines are highly effective in control. We know the story of poliomyelitis.

Today we are discussing a third general group of infections. These are infections due to organisms that are endogenous to the host and therefore are not very much influenced by environment. These are organisms intrinsic in the host in which the balance changes continuously between the host and the organism. It is in this group that we can expect to see future infectious disease problems arise and it is here that we know remarkably little about mechanisms of resistance and of production of disease.

However, although we have seen enormous changes occurring in etiology of infection within the hospital, we have yet no conclusive evidence that these changes also occur outside the hospital with anything even approaching the same magnitude. We are not certain whether the problem of the endogenous flora is one that is destined to replace other infectious disease problems, in a more general way, or whether this is a problem which is largely limited to the most susceptible population, which will end up in the hospital for one reason or another.

I am not trying to minimize the importance of the hospital infection problem but I do think that what we now need are base-line data which will give us a basis for comparing through the years, whether coliform infections or staphylococcic infections are truly increasing in a population in which we control for the other variables, and at present we do not have good data on this point. Therefore the question of whether opportunistic organisms are important outside of the special situations that pertain in hospitals must remain unanswered, and cannot be answered unless we start getting baseline data from large populations.

We can, for example, show that we can eliminate the staphylococcus from people with chronic bronchitis, but we cannot show yet that we are extending life in a significant way, because there is a high replacement with gram-negative rods. We can eliminate the Pseudomonas from the anaesthesia apparatus and lower the rate of Pseudomonas-related pulmonary disease, but have we lowered the total rate of chronic pulmonary disease ? Is the Pseudomonas implanted only in those people who are already susceptible to pulmonary infection ? It is this type of question which we must soon begin to answer. So far, in the field of hospital epidemiology, I can be clear about two findings. The first is that the inlying catheter, put into the bladder, produces disease and sometimes death, in people who were otherwise not likely to have this happen; secondly that the intravenous catheter does exactly the same thing. Under controlled conditions these complications can be prevented to some degree at least. These two examples are the only two in hospital epidemiology which I am prepared to accept as controlled, acceptable studies. The rest of it is more speculative and that is an unhappy admission which we must face and which must guide us to be more effective in our future investigations.

Reference

FINLAND, M.: The present status of antibiotics in bacterial infections. Bull. N. Y. Acad. Med. 27, 199—220 (1951).

Author Index

Names of principal speakers are set in **boldface,** those of speakers in discussions in *italics.*,
Figures in *italics* are references to the literature

Subject Index

GPSR Compliance
The European Union's (EU) General Product Safety Regulation (GPSR) is a set
of rules that requires consumer products to be safe and our obligations to
ensure this.

If you have any concerns about our products, you can contact us on

ProductSafety@springernature.com

In case Publisher is established outside the EU, the EU authorized
representative is:

Springer Nature Customer Service Center GmbH
Europaplatz 3
69115 Heidelberg, Germany